中医临床

中医临床

The Clinical Practice of Chinese Medicine

Psoriasis & Cutaneous Pruritus

by **Lu Chuan-jian**

Chief Physician & Professor of Chinese External Medicine, vice-President of the Second Teaching Hospital of Guangzhou University of CM, Guangzhou, China

Xuan Guo-wei

Chief Physician & Professor of Chinese External Medicine, the Second Teaching Hospital of Guangzhou University of CM, Guangzhou, China

Contributors

Hu Dong-liu, Associate Chief Physician

Huang Liang, M.S. TCM

Wang Lei, M.S. TCM

Wu Wei, M.S. TCM

Chi Feng-hao, Associate Chief Physician

Translated by

Zhou Ling, M.S. TCM & **Liu En-zhao**, M.S. TCM

Edited by

Douglas Darwin Eisenstark, L.Ac.

人民卫生出版社
PEOPLE'S MEDICAL PUBLISHING HOUSE

人民卫生出版社

PMPH PEOPLE´S MEDICAL PUBLISHING HOUSE

Website: http://www.pmph.com

Book Title: The Clinical Practice of Chinese Medicine:
Psoriasis & Cutaneous Pruritus
中医临床实用系列：银屑病与皮肤瘙痒症

Contact address: Bldg 3, 3 Qu, Fang Qun Yuan, Fang Zhuang, Beijing 100078, P. R. China, Phone/fax: 86 10 6761 7315, E-mail: pmph@pmph.com

Disclaimer

This book is for educational and reference purposes only. In view of the possibility of human error or changes in medical science, neither the author, editor nor the publisher nor any other party who has been involved in the preparation or publication of this work guarantees that the information contained herein is in every respect accurate or complete. The medicinal therapy and treatment techniques presented in this book are provided for the purpose of reference only. If readers wish to attempt any of the techniques or utilize any of the medicinal therapies contained in this book, the publisher assumes no responsibility for any such actions.

It is the responsibility of the readers to understand and adhere to local laws and regulations concerning the practice of these techniques and methods. The authors, editors and publishers disclaim all responsibility for any liability, loss, injury, or damage incurred as a consequence, directly or indirectly, of the use and application of any of the contents of this book.

First published: 2007
ISBN: 978-7-117-09242-5/R • 9243

Cataloguing in Publication Data:
A catalog record for this book is available from the CIP-Database China.

Printed in P.R. China

ISBN 978-7-117-09242-5

9 787117 092425 >

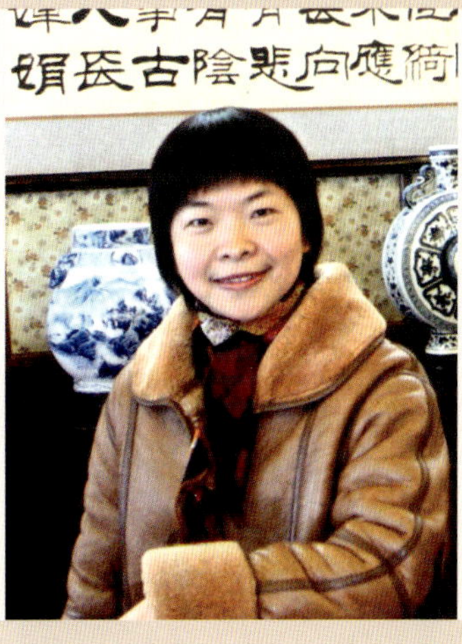

卢传坚 教授

Professor **Lu Chuan-jian** was born in October 1964. She is a Medical Doctor, professor, and state-approved Master's level Supervisor at the Second Teaching Hospital of Guangzhou University of Chinese Medicine (also known as the Guangdong Provincial Hospital of TCM). She is also the vice-president of this hospital. In addition, she serves as the vice-president of the Chinese Medicine Diagnosis Specialty Board of the Guangdong Provincial Medicine Association, the standing Director of Clinical Education Board of Advanced Education of Chinese Medicine Association, and as a member of the Dermatology Board of the Guangdong Provincial Medicine Association. She was chosen to be a successor of a famous senior physician Professor Shen Yan-nan in the national Master and Apprentice Education Program.

Through her years of clinical practice, teaching, and scientific research, she has achieved great curative effects in treating diseases such as psoriasis, eczema, urticaria, cutaneous pruritus, and herpes zoster. She has participated in 11 projects of scientific research on the national, provincial and bureau levels, and has published more than 50 research papers in national or provincial medical journals, as well as the monograph *Modern-day Treatment to Dermatology & Venereology*. She is the chief editor of *Urticaria, Eczema & Atopic Dermatitis*, and *Psoriasis & Cutaneous Pruritus*, as part of *the Clinical*

Practice of Chinese Medicine series. Professor Lu also participated in the editing and publication of *Diagnosis of Chinese Medicine* and *Collection of Cases in Dermatology*. She has won 7 clinical and teaching achievement awards.

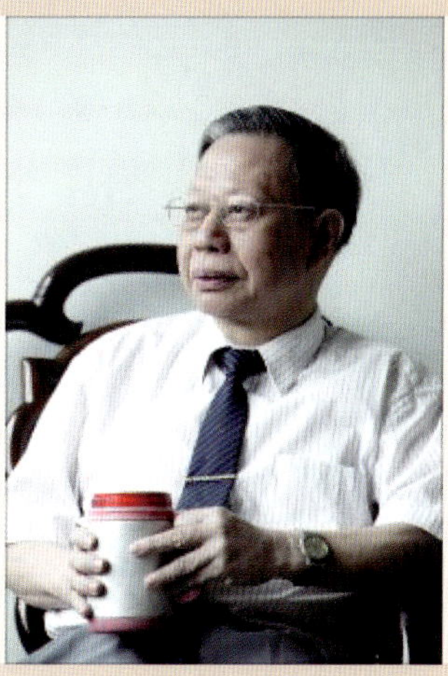

禤国维　教授

Professor **Xuan Guo-wei** serves as a professor, chief physician, and state-approved Doctoral Supervisor of the Guangzhou University of Chinese Medicine. He has also been given the title of "National Famous Physician of Chinese Medicine". As an expert, he has earned national recognition and is assigned as a Master Physician of the National Master and Apprentice Education Program. He was also the former director of the department of Dermatology and STD in Guangdong Provincial Hospital of TCM, consultant for the *Journal of Guangzhou University of Traditional Chinese Medicine*, as well as member of the editorial board for the *New Journal of Traditional Chinese Medicine*. Professor Xuan also serves as a consultant for the following societies: China Association of Chinese Medicine—Dermatology Board, Chinese Association of the Integration of Traditional and Western Medicine—Specialty Board for Dermatology and STD, and Guangdong Association of the Integration of Traditional and Western Medicine—Specialty Board for Dermatology and STD. He is the lifetime director of Guangdong Provincial Chinese Medicine Association and the honorary director of Guangdong Provincial Specialty Board for Dermatology and External Application of Chinese Medicine. In addition, he is a committee member of Guangdong Provincial and Guangzhou Municipal Special Board for Chinese medicine.

He has been engaged in clinical practice, teaching, and scientific research for more than 40 years. Over his long career in clinical practice, he has developed the special clinical approach—"tonifying the Kidney"—which is based on the principle of harmonizing yin and yang. The approach has been proved effective in the treatment of complicated dermatological diseases. Naturally, he is widely sought out by patients for treating difficult dermatological cases.

Professor Xuan has published over 60 research papers in several famous Chinese medicine journals, such as *Harmony of Yin and Yang as the Primary Treatment Principle* and *Insights of Clinical Diagnosis and Treatment of Dermatology*. He has edited 5 monographs including *Chinese Medicine Treatment of Dermatology and STD*, *Clinical Diagnosis and Treatment of Dermatology and STD in Chinese Medicine*. He co-authored the widely-used textbook of *Chinese External Medicine*. More recently, he took charge of 8 research projects at ministry and provincial levels. He has won several clinical and scientific research achievement awards at national and provincial levels.

Foreword

Chinese medicine is a broad and profound art of healing. It is a well-established and comprehensive system of medicine with an ancient origin and a long rich history. Throughout the ages, it has made a significant contribution to the prosperity of the Chinese civilization. The system of pattern differentiation and treatment fully reflects the Chinese medical view of health and disease as a holistic concept, the emphasis on the body's ability to regulate itself and adapt to the environment, and the need for individualized treatment. The integration of diseases and syndromes is the consummation of treatment based on pattern differentiation; it fully displays the superior characteristic of this discipline, and has an extensive influence on the development of the art of Chinese medicine.

The intention of this series of books is to introduce accurate Chinese medical diagnosis and treatment of various diseases to overseas readers.

The Chinese edition of *The Clinical Practice of Chinese Medicine* was edited by the Second Teaching Hospital of Guangzhou University of CM (also known as Guangdong Provincial Hospital of TCM), and published by People's Medical Publishing House. When the series was published in 2000, it was widely accepted in clinical practice due to its originality, distinguishing features, richness in content, completeness, accuracy, and outstanding emphases. This series has become a trademark of standard in the eyes of Chinese and integrative medical practitioners. During the second printing of this series of books, Professor Deng Tie-tao praised, "For a series to be printed a multiple number of times, shows that it is highly regarded and has received excellent reviews." In order to keep up with the constant development of medical science, this series was revised and re-published in 2004 by People's Medical Publishing House. Due to its popularity, it has been reprinted numerous times since.

The English edition of this series of books includes 20 volumes:

- *COPD & Asthma*
- *Coronary Artery Disease & Hyperlipidemia*
- *Stroke & Parkinson's Disease*
- *Chronic Gastritis & Irritable Bowel Syndrome*
- *Diabetes & Obesity*
- *Gout & Rheumatoid Arthritis*
- *Menstrual Disorders I: Dysfunctional Uterine Bleeding & Amenorrhea*
- *Menstrual Disorders II: Premenstrual Syndrome, Dysmenorrhea & Perimenopause*
- *Endometriosis & Uterine Fibroids*
- *Pelvic Inflammatory Disease & Miscarriage*
- *Postpartum Hypogalactia & Breast Hyperplasia*
- *Male & Female Infertility*
- *Urticaria*
- *Eczema & Atopic Dermatitis*
- *Lupus Erythematosus*
- *Scleroderma & Dermatomyositis*
- *Diseases of the Accessory Organs of the Skin*
- *Psoriasis & Cutaneous Pruritus*
- *Herpes Zoster & Fungal Skin Infections*
- *Chloasma & Vitiligo*

Clinical application varies by individual and by location; when this is combined with the rapid development of medical science, the treatment methods and medicinal dosages may also vary accordingly. When using these books as a reference guide, overseas readers should confirm the formulas and dosages of medicinals according to the individual health condition of the patient, as well as take into account the origin of the Chinese medicinals.

The quotes in these books were taken from various medical literature during the compilation process. We have deleted some of the contents of the original texts for the purpose of uniformity and ease in readability. We ask for the reader's forgiveness and express our respect and gratitude toward the original authors.

Due to the complicated nature of the diagnoses and treatments covered in these books, and the wide range of topics they touch upon, it is inevitable that one may encounter errors while reading through them. We respectively welcome constructive criticism and corrections from our readers.

The clinical practice of medicine changes with the constant development of medical science. The books in this series will be revised regularly to continuously adapt to the development of traditional Chinese medicine.

Editorial Board for the English edition of
The Clinical Practice of Chinese Medicine series
September, 2007

Editorial Board

for the English edition of

The Clinical Practice of Chinese Medicine Series

Wu Xian-zhong

Specialist of Integrative Medicine, Academician of Chinese Academy of Engineering, Professor, Tianjin Medical University, Chairman of Tianjin Institute of Acute Abdomen Research on Integrative Medicine

Wang Yong-yan

Specialist of Chinese Internal Medicine, Academician of Chinese Academy of Engineering, Professor and former President of Beijing University of CM, and Honorary President of China Academy of Chinese Medical Science

Chen Ke-ji

Specialist of Cardiovascular & Aging Diseases, Academician of Chinese Academy of Science, Professor of Medicine, Xiyuan Hospital, and Institute of Aging Medicine, China Academy of Chinese Medical Science, Consultant on Traditional Medicine, WHO

General Coordinator

Lü Yu-bo

Professor & Vice President, Guangzhou University of CM,
President, the Second Teaching Hospital of Guangzhou University of CM

Editors-in-Chief

Luo Yun-jian

Guangdong Province Entitled Famous Chinese Medicine Physician,Professor of Chinese Internal Medicine, & former Vice President of the Second Teaching Hospital of Guangzhou University of CM

Liu Mao-cai

Guangdong Province Entitled Famous Chinese Medicine Physician,Professor of Chinese Internal Medicine, & former Vice President of the Second Teaching Hospital of Guangzhou University of CM, Former Chairman of Institute for Aging Cerebral Diseases, Guangzhou University of CM

Associate Editors-in-Chief

Xuan Guo-wei

Guangdong Province Entitled Famous Chinese Medicine Physician, Director & Professor, Department of Chinese External Medicine, Guangzhou University of CM, Former Vice President of the Second Teaching Hospital of Guangzhou University of CM

Huang Chun-lin

Professor of Chinese Internal Medicine, & former Associate-Director of the Second Institute for Clinical Research, Guangzhou University of CM

Chen Da-can

Professor of Chinese External Medicine, Vice President of the Second Teaching Hospital of Guangzhou University of CM

Chen Zhi-qiang

Professor of Chinese External Medicine, Director of the Department of Surgery, Vice President of the Second Teaching Hospital of Guangzhou University of CM

Feng Wei-bin

Professor of Chinese Internal Medicine, the Second Teaching Hospital of Guangzhou University of CM

Yang Zhi-min

Professor of Chinese Internal Medicine, Vice President of the Second Teaching Hospital of Guangzhou University of CM

Lu Chuan-jian

Professor of Chinese External Medicine, Vice President of the Second Teaching Hospital of Guangzhou University of CM

Zou Xu

Professor of Chinese Internal Medicine, Vice President of the Second Teaching Hospital of Guangzhou University of CM

Members (Listed alphabetically by name)

Deng Zhao-zhi

Professor of Chinese Internal Medicine, Guangzhou University of CM

Fan Guan-jie

Professor of Chinese Internal Medicine, Director of Department of Education, the Second Teaching Hospital of Guangzhou University of CM

Fan Rui-qiang

Professor of Chinese External Medicine, Director of Department of Dermatology, the Second Teaching Hospital of Guangzhou University of CM

Huang Jian-ling

Professor of Chinese Medicine Gynecology, Director of the First Department of Gynecology, the Second Teaching Hospital of Guangzhou University of CM

Huang Pei-xin

Professor of Chinese Internal Medicine, the Second Teaching Hospital of Guangzhou University of CM, Head of the Research Project of Cerebral Disease Treatment on Chinese Internal Medicine, Sponsored by SATCM China

Huang Sui-ping

Professor of Chinese Internal Medicine, Director of Department of Digestion, the Second Teaching Hospital of Guangzhou University of CM

Li Li-yun

Guangdong Province Entitled Famous Chinese Medicine Physician, Professor of Chinese Medicine Gynecology, the Second Teaching Hospital of Guangzhou University of CM

Liang Xue-fang

Professor of Chinese Medicine Gynecology, Director of the Third Department of Gynecology, the Second Teaching Hospital of Guangzhou University of CM

Lin Lin

Professor of Chinese Internal Medicine, Director of Department of Respiratory, the Second Teaching Hospital of Guangzhou University of CM

Lin Yi

Professor of Mastopathy in Chinese Medicine, the Second Teaching Hospital of Guangzhou University of CM, Head of the National Key Subject –Mastopathy in Chinese Medicine

Liu Wei-sheng

Master of the National Master and Apprentice Education Program, Professor of Chinese Internal Medicine, the Second Teaching Hospital of Guangzhou University of CM

Si-tu Yi

Professor of Chinese Medicine Gynecology, the Second Teaching Hospital of Guangzhou University of CM, Head of the National Key Subject – Chinese Medicine Gynecology

Wang Xiao-yun

Professor of Chinese Medicine Gynecology, Director of Department of Gynecology, Head of Teaching Division of Gynecology, the Second Teaching Hospital of Guangzhou University of CM

Sponsored by

The Second Teaching Hospital of Guangzhou University of CM,
also known as **Guangdong Provincial Hospital of TCM**

Preface

Dermatology is a significant component of traditional Chinese medicine and has an exceedingly rich content due to the accumulation of several thousand years of valuable clinical experience. In the last ten years, there have been especially encouraging developments in the use of traditional Chinese medicine, Western medicine and integrative medicine for the treatment of difficult skin disorders such as eczema, psoriasis, vitiligo, and hair loss. There have also been successes with clear clinical curative effects, leading to international standards.

The authors of this series are all Chinese medical doctors who have abundant clinical knowledge through years of practicing dermatology, as well as having published many dermatology text books. Through this compilation process, we have tried to give a detailed introduction to TCM syndrome differentiation and treatments. We have consulted with dermatology specialists to collect advice and suggestions, as well as to summarize their experience with effective treatments. We have also referenced a large number of related national and international documents that analyze and explore the subject based on current research results. This series is a summarization and refinement of the clinical treatment of skin diseases with Chinese medicine. It is also our thorough reflection on the most salient points and challenges of this subject.

Psoriasis and cutaneous pruritus are commonly seen in the dermatology department. Psoriasis affects people's appearance and brings patients important physical and mental harm. Due to its lingering course, it is referred to as a "non-fatal-survivable cancer". However, the complex etiological factors of cutaneous pruritus increase the difficulties of treatment. The antipruritic therapies of biomedicine achieve good curative effects but with various side effects. Researchers and clinicians around the world have been giving increased attention to the treatment of these disorders. While biomedicine can have good therapeutic effects, they are not extensively applied clinically due to the severe side effects. On the other hand, Chinese medicine has obvious effective treatment to relieve and control pathological conditions by classifying them according to the complete system of pattern differentiation, and applying effective treatments according to different clinical manifestations.

In this series of books, readers will find an organized and thorough presentation of each disease, including a brief overview, etiology, pathomechanism, various Chinese medical treatment modalities, prognosis, preventive healthcare practices, case studies, comments from famous physicians, integrative treatment approaches, quotes from classical texts, and modern research.

The brief overview offers a general introduction to the biomedical view of the disease.

Discussions of etiology, pathomechanism, and Chinese medical treatment are from the perspective of Chinese medicine, and reflect upon the onset, diagnosis, pattern differentiation, and treatment of the disease.

Cases and comments from many famous physicians are collected in the section of the clinical experience of renowned physicians.

The chapter on integrative treatment approaches emphasizes the advantages of Chinese medical treatments, as well as discussing the proper time for the intervention of biomedicine. To the Western reader, this section presents clear mode of thinking in terms of the integration of Chinese medicine and biomedicine.

Quotes from classical texts and modern research provide abundant references on these diseases.

This series of books present a clear description of each disease as well as the key points for diagnosis and treatment using Chinese medicine.

These books discuss, in detail, the clinical experience of ancient and modern-day renowned physicians, thereby enabling the practitioner to become more adept at using Chinese medicine in the diagnosis and treatment of common diseases.

In order to ensure a better understanding of the contents of this Chinese medical book series, we have recognized that different readers have different needs and expectations.

First, medical professionals, practitioners and students, who read this series for professional study and application should have a solid background in the basic theory of Chinese medicine, as well as a command of the ingredients and indications of classical formulas. Prior to reading this book, they should also know the properties of herbs and combination contraindications. When using the herbs in clinic, practitioners should note the doses of medicinals and their place of origin. It is important that in countries without a Chinese herbal medicine tradition, to have a deep understanding of the functions and incompatibilities of the herbs. On this basis, one can choose to substitute similar medicinals and formulas to treat illness.

Second, readers who are interested in Chinese medicine should note the characteristics and advantages of Chinese medicine, and the special methods of Chinese medicine in the areas of prognosis and preventive healthcare. When treating patients, if similar symptoms occur, medicine should be prescribed only under the guidance of professional Chinese medical physicians.

We hope that these books will prove to be useful and valuable to all of those involved in the field of Chinese medicine, including practitioners, students, teachers, patients, medical doctors who are interested in Chinese medicine, and anyone who may be seeking answers to their questions about the efficacy of Chinese medicine. Hopefully, this book can help readers gain a deeper understanding of Chinese medical diagnosis and treatment in the field of dermatology, as well as build a bridge between Chinese medicine and biomedicine through the discussion of integrative treatment approaches.

Due to the nature of clinical medicine, we apologize for any outdated or incorrect information that may appear in these books. We hope that readers will not hesitate to offer their comments and suggestions on how to improve the content of this material.

Lu Chuan-jian & Xuan Guo-wei
Guangzhou China
September 2007

Contents

Cutaneous Pruritus 083

Psoriasis

by **Lu Chuan-jian**, Professor & Chief Physician of Chinese External Medicine
Hu Dong-liu, Associate Chief Physician of Chinese External Medicine
Wu Wei, M.S. TCM
Huang Liang, M.S. TCM

OVERVIEW

Psoriasis is a common chronic recurrent inflammatory skin disease characterized by special skin damage, called neurodermatitis. It manifests clinically as red papules or plaque covered with layers of dry silver scales (argentate squamae) or small, inflamed, pus-filled, blister-like lesions on the surface of the skin (pustules). Psoriasis mainly occurs on the lateral sides of the limbs, scalp and back.

According to its clinical features, psoriasis is classified into several categories, including: an ordinary pattern, agria (pustule) pattern, arthropathia (arthritic) pattern or an erythrodermia (redness) pattern.

The basic damage of the ordinary pattern is most commonly seen as inflammatory red papules or maculopapule covered with layers of dry argentate squamae.

The three major clinical features of psoriasis are white scaling (squamae), glazing membrane (shiny) and punctate hemorrhage (dots of blood).

During the progression of the disease, there are varieties of skin damage which are mostly seen on the scalp and the lateral aspects of the limbs and nails. Depending on the development of the patient's condition, it is classified as either the active phase, stable phase or the remission phase.

Pustule psoriasis is relatively rare and is classified into either the general pattern or the metacarpus (hand) and metatarsus (foot) pattern. It manifests as a superficial concentration of uninfected small pustules ranging from pinhead to a millet size.

Arthritic psoriasis is commonly seen and manifests anywhere in the body with a skin rash. There is red swelling and aching in the joints on exertion, morning stiffness and limitations on activities. In this way it resembles rheumatoid arthritis.

Erythrodermic psoriasis is commonly seen and is frequently caused by improper treatment of ordinary psoriasis or after the subsidence of pustule psoriasis. Exfoliative dermatitis can be seen extending over the entire body with diffuse red or dark red skin and obvious inflammatory infiltration covered by large areas of scaling that looks like wheat bran.

Biomedicine practitioners do not yet completely understand the etiology and pathomechanisms of psoriasis. At present, it is generally thought that psoriasis can be due to hereditary factors, infections, metabolic dysfunctions, endocrine influences, immune issues and many kinds of nervous system factors. These then influence various kinds of epidemic cell hyperplasia, incomplete keratinization and inflammatory reactions.

The diagnostic feature of ordinary psoriasis is erythema and papules that are covered by many layers of silvery-white argentate squamae. Scraping reveals a layer of pink semitransparent membranes called the "membrane phenomenon". When the membrane is again scraped, small pink bleeding points appear. These are called either the "punctate hemorrhage phenomenon" or also called the "isomorphic effect". There may also be an effect of pitted "thimble fingernails". The onset begins in young people in the prime of their life and progresses slowly. It is seasonal, being heavier in winter and lighter in summer. The pathology changes its nature to one of incomplete keratinization. Munro abscesses (microscopic white blood cells on the skin surface) can be identified.

Psoriasis is a recurrent, chronic inflammatory disease with various causative factors. Although it can not be cured completely, through proper treatment, with new therapies and drugs, the pathogenic condition can be relieved and to a great extent patient's lives can be improved. The treatment varies according to type, skin damage, distributing area, age and concurrent diseases.

At present, the treatment strategies include: control the pathogenic condition as quickly as possible, sustain the longest remission time and reduce drug side effects as much as possible. For biomedical treatment, antineoplastic agents, immune depressants, retinoid and corticosteroids are generally prescribed. Drugs for external use are usually cutin exfoliative agents, cell-directed inhibitors and reducing agents.

When covering a wound, first wash the scales (squamae) with soap and warm water. In the acute phase do not use strong stimulating medications that may induce inflammation. For cases of effusion, treat it as if it were an acute or subacute inflammation. At the beginning, prescribe medications with a low potency. Then use discretion before moving to a higher potency.

Psoriasis belongs to *Bai Bi* (white crust) in Chinese medicine.

CHINESE MEDICAL ETIOLOGY AND PATHOMECHANISM

Practitioners of Chinese medicine believe that psoriasis is caused by a combination of exterior and interior pathogens. There may be heat accumulation obstructing the blood vessels due to an external invasion, impairment of the seven emotions (affects) and/or a disharmony of the spleen and stomach.

1. Invasion of Exogenous Pathogens

The beginning of the disease is often caused by a qi and blood disharmony due to an invasion of wind, damp, heat or fire toxins on the skin obstructing the pores and interstitial spaces. It can also be caused by a damp-heat accumulation unable to eliminate internally (through the urine or bowels) or externally (through perspiration) because of exterior blockage. Psoriasis can also be caused by a chronic disease which consumes qi and blood that then fails to nourish the skin.

2. Impairment of the Seven Emotions

Because of the constraint of emotions (affects), the regulation and the movement of qi become obstructed and then eventually transforms into fire. This fire changes to fire toxins which then accumulate in the nutritive blood. When these toxins flow to the muscles and skin, then psoriasis is created.

3. Disharmony of Spleen and Stomach

An improper and excessive diet of fish and wind-stirring foods causes a disharmony of the Spleen and Stomach. This creates qi stagnation and damp-heat accumulation that becomes obstructed in the skin that in turn creates psoriasis.

In addition, some patients suffer from improper medical treatment and suffer infections from toxic pathogens. Heat toxins flow into the nutritive blood level causing scorching heat that involves both the qi and blood. This heat then consumes yin and blood. In chronic illness, qi and blood stagnation in the meridians and collaterals can cause skin to become thick and hardened.

CHINESE MEDICAL TREATMENT

To treat psoriasis, various therapies are prescribed both externally and internally according to the clinical manifestations, typing and staging.

Pattern Differentiation and Treatment

Clinical syndrome differentiations at the earlier stage of psoriasis are primarily excess syndromes such as blood-heat, damp-heat, wind-heat and fire toxins. At the intermediate stage, the syndrome is usually a blood deficiency-wind dryness pattern. At the advanced stage, it often is a blood stasis pattern. Psoriatic arthritis is often seen as a wind-damp-cold *bi* syndrome (painful syndrome) .

1. Wind-heat and Blood-heat

【Syndrome Characteristics】

Skin damage continuously increasing, sensation of itching, usually aggravated in summer, accompanied by aversion to heat, brownish urination and dry stool. Red tongue with thin yellow coating, slippery and rapid pulse.

【Treatment Principle】

Expel wind and eliminate heat, cool blood and remove ecchymoses (escape of blood under the skin).

【Commonly Used Medicinals】

To cool blood and remove ecchymoses, use *shuǐ niú jiǎo* (Cornu Bubali), *bái máo gēn* (Rhizoma Imperatae), *mǔ dān pí* (Cortex Moutan), *zǐ cǎo* (Radix Arnebiae), *bái xiān pí* (Cortex Dictamni) and *shēng dì huáng* (Radix Rehmanniae Recens). To dispel wind and relieve itching, use *jīng jiè* (Herba Schizonepetae), *fáng fēng* (Radix Saposhnikoviae) and *chán tuì* (Periostracum Cicadae).

【Representative Formula】

Modified *Xiāo Fēng Sǎn* with *Xī Jiǎo Dì Huáng Tāng* (消风散合犀角地黄汤).

【Ingredients】

荆芥	jīng jiè	9g	Herba Schizonepetae
防风	fáng fēng	9g	Radix Saposhnikoviae
生地黄	shēng dì huáng	15g	Radix Rehmanniae Recens
水牛角	shuǐ niú jiǎo	50g	Cornu Bubali
赤芍	chì sháo	15g	Radix Paeoniae Rubra
牡丹皮	mǔ dān pí	9g	Cortex Moutan
苦参	kǔ shēn	15g	Radix Sophorae Flavescentis
知母	zhī mǔ	9g	Rhizoma Anemarrhenae
生石膏	shēng shí gāo	30g	Gypsum Fivrosum
通草	tōng cǎo	9g	Medulla Tetrapanacis
蝉蜕	chán tuì	6g	Periostracum Cicadae

牛蒡子	niú bàng zǐ	15g	Fructus Arctii
甘草	gān cǎo	6g	Radix et Rhizoma Glycyrrhizae

Combine the above Chinese medicinals in 500ml of water, simmer down to 100ml, divide in half and drink warm twice a day.

【Formula Analysis】

Jīng jiè (Herba Schizonepetae) and *fáng fēng* (Radix Saposhnikoviae) are used as the chief herbs to expel wind and relieve the exterior. *Shēng dì huáng* (Radix Rehmanniae Recens), *shuǐ niú jiǎo* (Cornu Bubali), *chì sháo* (Radix Paeoniae Rubra) and *mǔ dān pí* (Cortex Moutan) are used as deputies to enter into the *Xue Fen* (blood level) to cool blood and remove ecchymoses, dispel wind and relieve itching. *Zhī mǔ* (Rhizoma Anemarrhenae) and *shí gāo* (Gypsum Fivrosum) are used as assistants for clearing heat to reduce fire. *Tōng cǎo* (Medulla Tetrapanacis) clearing heat by diuresis and is used as the envoy.

【Modifications】

- To relieve sore-throat and resolve toxins, add *dà qīng yè* (Folium Isatidis) 15g and *zhè bèi mǔ* (Bulbus Fritillariae Thunbergii) 15g.
- For dry stool and constipation, add *dà huáng* (Radix et Rhizoma Rhei) (decoct later) 9g, *hòu pò* (Cortex Magnoliae Officinalis) 15g and *zhǐ shí* (Fructus Aurantii Immaturus) 15g, to clear heat from the *fu* organs.

2. Blood Deficiency and Wind Dryness

【Syndrome Characteristics】

This is a stable condition with no enlargement of the eruptions or few new ones. There is dry skin (perhaps with lichenation) on the front and sides of the calfs of the legs. Possibly chapping in the lateral creases of the joints, painful, sometimes accompanied by dizziness and blurred eyes, pale and weak complexion. The tongue is pale with a thin coating and a thin, soggy pulse.

【Treatment Principle】

Enrich blood to moist dryness, dispel wind to relieve itching.

【Commonly Used Medicinals】

To enrich blood and moisten dryness, use *dāng guī* (Radix Angelicae Sinensis), *shǒu wū* (Radix Polygoni Multiflori), *shēng dì huáng* (Radix Rehmanniae Recens), *bái sháo* (Raidix Paeoniae Alba), *xuán shēn* (Raidix Scrophulariae) and *mài dōng* (Raidix Ophiopogonis). To relieve itching by dispelling wind, use *jiāng cán* (Bombyx Batryticatus) and *chán tuì* (Periostracum Cicadae).

【Representative Formula】

Modified *Yǎng Xuè Qū Fēng Rùn Fū Tāng* (养血祛风润肤汤).

【Ingredients】

当归	dāng guī	9g	Radix Angelicae Sinensis
熟地黄	shú dì huáng	15g	Radix Rehmanniae Praeparata
天门冬	tiān mén dōng	9g	Radix Asparagi
麦门冬	mài mén dōng	9g	Raidix Ophiopogonis
生黄芪	shēng huáng qí	20g	Radix Astragali (raw)
桃仁	táo rén	9g	Semen Persicae
红花	hóng huā	6g	Flos Carthami
黄芩	huáng qín	10g	Radix Scutellariae
天花粉	tiān huā fěn	9g	Radix Trichosanthis
甘草	gān cǎo	6g	Radix et Rhizoma Glycyrrhizae

Combine the above Chinese medicinals in 500ml of water and decoct to 100ml. Divide the decoction in half and take twice a day.

【Formula Analysis】

Dāng guī (Radix Angelicae Sinensis) and *shú dì huáng* (Radix Rehmanniae Praeparata) are used to enrich blood and moisten dryness as the chief herbs. *Shēng huáng qí* (raw Radix Astragali) tonifying qi and generating blood, *tiān mén dōng* (Radix Asparagi) and *mài mén dōng* (Raidix Ophiopogonis) benefiting yin and moistening dryness are used together as the deputies. *Táo rén* (Semen Persicae) and *hóng huā* (Flos Carthami) invigorating blood, *huáng qín* (Radix Scutellariae) and *tiān huā fěn* (Radix Trichosanthis) clearing heat and generating fluids are used as assistants.

【Modifications】

➢ For dysphoria (vexation and agitation) and insomnia, add *suān zǎo rén* (Semen Ziziphi Spinosae) 12g and *yè jiāo téng* (Caulis Polygoni Multiflori) 15g to enrich the heart and calm the mind.

➢ For dry mouth and throat, subtract *shēng huáng qí* (raw Radix Astragali), and add *shí gāo* (Gypsum Fibrosum) (decoct first) 30g and *zhī mǔ* (Rhizoma Anemarrhenae) 15g to clear heat and generate fluids to remove agitation.

3. Damp-heat Accumulation

【Syndrome Characteristics】

Damp-heat accumulation is usually seen in the armpit and inguinal fold. There may be erosive erythema with pustular fluid effusion and itching in the palms and soles of the hands and feet. It is aggravated on cloudy and rainy days and may be accompanied by chest oppression and with a loss of appetite, exhaustion, heavy limbs or profuse yellow leucorrhea. There is a thin, yellow and greasy tongue coat, and a soggy and slippery pulse.

【Treatment Principle】

Clear heat and eliminate dampness, cool blood and remove areas of bleeding under the skin (ecchymoses).

【Commonly Used Medicinals】

To clear heat and eliminate dampness, use *jīn yín huā* (Flos Lonicerae), *bì xiè* (Rhizoma Dioscoreae Hypoglaucae), *tǔ fú líng* (Rhizoma Smilacis Glabrae), *yì yǐ rén* (Semen Coicis), *zé xiè* (Rhizoma Alismatis) and *chē qián zǐ* (Semen Plantaginis). To cool blood and remove ecchymoses, use *dān pí* (Cortex Moutan), *chì sháo* (Radix Paeoniae Rubra) and *shēng dì huáng* (Radix Rehmanniae Recens).

【Representative Formula】

Modified *Bì Xiè Shèn Shī Tāng* (萆薢渗湿汤).

【Ingredients】

萆薢	bì xiè	9g	Rhizoma Dioscoreae Hypoglaucae
黄柏	huáng bǎi	9g	Cortex Phellodendri
泽泻	zé xiè	15g	Rhizoma Alismatis
薏苡仁	yì yǐ rén	30g	Semen Coicis
滑石	huá shí	20g	Talcum
通草	tōng cǎo	10g	Medulla Tetrapanacis
车前子	chē qián zǐ	15g	Semen Plantaginis
赤芍	chì sháo	15g	Radix Paeoniae Rubra
牡丹皮	mǔ dān pí	9g	Cortex Moutan
甘草	gān cǎo	6g	Radix et Rhizoma Glycyrrhizae

Combine the above Chinese medicinals in 500ml water, decoct to 100ml and divide in half to drink twice a day while the decoction is warm.

【Formula Analysis】

Bì xiè (Rhizoma Dioscoreae Hypoglaucae), *huáng bǎi* (Cortex Phellodendri), *zé xiè* (Rhizoma Alismatis), *yì yǐ rén* (Semen Coicis) and *huá shí* (Talcum) are used as the chief herbs to clear heat and eliminate dampness. *Tōng cǎo* (Medulla Tetrapanacis) and *chē qián zǐ* (Semen Plantaginis) are used as deputies to clear heat and create diuresis. *Mǔ dān pí* (Cortex Moutan) and *chì sháo* (Radix Paeoniae Rubra) are used as assistants to cool blood and remove ecchymoses. *Gān cǎo* (Radix et Rhizoma Glycyrrhizae) is the envoy used to harmonize the rest of the herbs.

For extensive skin damage and pustules add medicinals such as *pú gōng yīng* (Herba Taraxaci) 30g, *tǔ fú líng* (Rhizoma Smilacis Glabrae) 30g and *rěn dōng téng* (Caulis Lonicerae) 30g to clear heat and resolve toxins.

4. Fire Toxin Flourishing

【Syndrome Characteristics】

The syndrome characteristics of fire toxin flourishing are redness on the skin over the entire body, or dark red and perhaps even slightly edematous swelling. There is relatively little scaling, burning sensations on the skin or densely scattered pustules. It can be accompanied by a strong fever and thirst, dry stool, brownish urine. The tongue is deep red/crimson with a thin coating and a wiry, slippery and rapid pulse.

【Treatment Principle】

Purge fire to cool blood and resolve foxins.

【Commonly Used Medicinals】

To purge fire and resolve foxins to remove ecchymoses use *huáng lián* (Rhizoma Coptidis), *huáng qín* (Radix Scutellariae), *yě jú huā* (Flos Chrysanthemi Indici), *shēng shí gāo* (Gypsum Fivrosum), *zhī zǐ* (Fructus Gardeniae) and *lián qiào* (Fructus Forsythiae). To cool blood and remove ecchymoses use *shuǐ niú jiǎo* (Cornu Bubali), *mǔ dān pí* (Cortex Moutan) and *shēng dì huáng* (Radix Rehmanniae Recens).

【Representative Medicinals】

Modified *Huáng Lián Jiě Dú Tāng* with *Wǔ Wèi Xiāo Dú Yǐn* (黄连解毒汤合五味消毒饮).

【Ingredients】

黄连	huáng lián	6g	Rhizoma Coptidis
黄柏	huáng bǎi	9g	Cortex Phellodendri
黄芩	huáng qín	12g	Radix Scutellariae
栀子	zhī zǐ	9g	Fructus Gardeniae
蒲公英	pú gōng yīng	20g	Herba Taraxaci
金银花	jīn yín huā	9g	Flos Lonicerae
野菊花	yě jú huā	15g	Flos Chrysanthemi Indici
天葵子	tiān kuí zǐ	9g	Radix Semiaquilegiae
紫花地丁	zǐ huā dì dīng	9g	Herba Violae
甘草	gān cǎo	6g	Radix et Rhizoma Glycyrrhizae

Combine all the above Chinese medicinals, to 500ml of water, decoct to 100ml, divide and drink warm twice a day.

【Formula Analysis】

Huáng lián (Rhizoma Coptidis), *huáng bǎi* (Cortex Phellodendri) and *huáng qín* (Radix Scutellariae) are used to purge fire in *San Jiao* and are the chief herbs. *Zhī zǐ* (Fructus Gardeniae) as the deputy is used to purge *San Jiao*. The assistants *jīn yín huā* (Flos Lonicerae), *tiān kuí zǐ* (Radix Semiaquilegiae), *yě jú huā* (Flos Chrysanthemi Indici) and *zǐ huā dì dīng* (Herba Violae) are used to clear heat to cool blood and resolve toxins. *Gān cǎo* (Radix et Rhizoma Glycyrrhizae) is used as the envoy to harmonize the other herbs. The whole prescription functions to purge fire, clear heat and resolve toxins.

【Modifications】

➢ For a strong fever, coma and irritability, take one pill of *Ān Gōng Niú Huáng Wán* (安宫牛黄丸) or *Zhì Bǎo Dān* (至宝丹) to open the orifices and clear heat and resolve toxins.

➢ For dry stool and constipation, add *dà huáng* (Radix et Rhizoma Rhei) (decoct later) 9g and *máng xiāo* (Natrii Sulfas) (take after mixing with decoction) to clear heat from the *fu* organs.

5. Blood Stasis

【Syndrome Characteristics】

Blood stasis is a prolonged, recurrent and obstinate pathogenic condition with dark purple skin damage or hyperpigmentation. There is thick scaling that may take on the texture of an oyster shell or accompanied by impaired joint mobility. The tongue may have stasis spots and a thin coating. The pulse is thready and rough.

【Treatment Principle】

Invigorate blood and transform stasis, enrich blood and moisten dryness.

【Commonly Used Medicinals】

To invigorate blood and transform stasis, use *táo rén* (Semen Persicae), *hóng huā* (Flos Carthami), *dān shēn* (Radix et Rhizoma Salviae

Miltiorrhizae), *niú xī* (Radix Acanthopanacis Bidentatae), *sān léng* (Rhizoma Sparganii) and *é zhú* (Rhizoma Curcumae). To enrich blood and moisten dryness, use *dāng guī* (Radix Angelicae Sinensis), *shēng dì huáng* (Radix Rehmanniae Recens) and *jī xuè téng* (Caulis Spatholobi).

【Representative Formula】

Modified *Táo Hóng Sì Wù Tāng* (桃红四物汤).

【Ingredients】

熟地黄	shú dì huáng	15g	Radix Rehmanniae Praeparata
当归	dāng guī	12g	Radix Angelicae Sinensis
桃仁	táo rén	9g	Semen Persicae
红花	hóng huā	6g	Flos Carthami
丹参	dān shēn	15g	Radix et Rhizoma Salviae Miltiorrhizae
赤芍	chì sháo	9g	Radix Paeoniae Rubra
川芎	chuān xiōng	15g	Rhizoma Chuanxiong
甘草	gān cǎo	6g	Radix et Rhizoma Glycyrrhizae

Combine the above Chinese medicinals in 500ml of water, simmer down to 100ml, divide in half and drink warm twice a day.

【Formula Analysis】

Use *dāng guī* (Radix Angelicae Sinensis) for tonifying and enriching blood and *shú dì huáng* (Radix Rehmanniae Praeparata) for tonifying blood as chief herbs. The deputies, *táo rén* (Semen Persicae) and *hóng huā* (Flos Carthami) enter the blood level to drive away stasis and promote blood circulation. They are used with *dān shēn* (Radix et Rhizoma Salviae Miltiorrhizae) to invigorate and tonify blood. *Chuān xiōng* (Rhizoma Chuanxiong) enters the blood level to promote qi circulation within the blood. *Chì sháo* (Radix Paeoniae Rubra) preserves yin to nourish the blood. Both are the assistants. *Gān cǎo* (Radix et Rhizoma Glycyrrhizae) is used as the envoy to harmonize the other medicinals.

【Modifications】

➢ For a severe pathogenic condition with dark purple skin damage and heavy blood stasis, add *sān léng* (Rhizoma Sparganii) 9g and *é zhú* (Rhizoma Curcumae) 9g to break up blood stasis.

6. Wind-damp and Cold Arthromyodynia

【Syndrome Characteristics】

This condition features a pale skin eruption with thick scales that are easy to dislodge when scratched. It often begins or is aggravated in the winter, and disappears in the summer. It can be accompanied by an aversion to cold, aching and painful joints, and itching. The tongue has a thin clear-white coating and a floating, soggy and slippery pulse.

【Treatment Principle】

Expel wind and remove cold, harmonize nutritive blood and unblock collaterals.

【Commonly Used Medicinals】

To expel wind and disperse cold, use *guì zhī* (Ramulus Cinnamomi), *chuān niú xī* (Radix Acanthopanacis Bidentatae), *fáng fēng* (Radix Saposhnikoviae) and *shēng jiāng* (Rhizoma Zingiberis Recens). To eliminate dampness and unblock collaterals, use *wēi líng xiān* (Radix et Rhizoma Clematidis), *dú huó* (Radix Angelicae Pubescentis) and *qín jiāo* (Radix Gentianae Macrophyllae).

【Representative Formula】

Modified *Guì Zhī Tāng* (桂枝汤).

【Ingredients】

桂枝	guì zhī	9g	Ramulus Cinnamomi
白芍	bái sháo	9g	Radix Paeoniae Rubra
苍耳子	cāng ěr zǐ	9g	Fructus Xanthii
白芷	bái zhǐ	9g	Radix Angelicae Dahuricae
白鲜皮	bái xiān pí	20g	Cortex Dictamni
地肤子	dì fū zǐ	9g	Fructus Kochiae
大枣	dà zǎo	10 pcs	Fructus Jujubae
当归	dāng guī	9g	Radix Angelicae Sinensis

炙甘草	zhì gān cǎo	6g	Radix et Rhizoma Glycyrrhizae Praeparata cum Melle
生姜	shēng jiāng	3 pcs	Rhizoma Zingiberis Recens

Combine the above Chinese medicinals in 500ml of water, simmer down to 100ml, divide in half and drink warm twice a day.

【Formula Analysis】

Chief herbs *guì zhī* (Ramulus Cinnamomi) expels wind and removes cold along with *bái sháo* (Radix Paeoniae) which coordinates nutritive blood and preserves yin. *Cāng ěr zǐ* (Fructus Xanthii), *bái zhǐ* (Radix Angelicae Dahuricae), *dì fū zǐ* (Fructus Kochiae) and *bái xiān pí* (Cortex Dictamni) are the deputies and dispel wind to relieve itching. *Dà zǎo* (Fructus Jujubae) and *dāng guī* (Radix Angelicae Sinensis) enrich blood and coordinate nutritive blood as assistants. *Shēng jiāng* (Rhizoma Zingiberis Recens) removes cold and with *gān cǎo* (Radix et Rhizoma Glycyrrhizae) harmonizes the other herbs (envoys).

【Modifications】

➢ For joint abnormity or dysfunction, add *qiāng huó* (Rhizoma et Radix Notopterygii) 10g, *dú huó* (Radix Angelicae Pubescentis) 10g, *sāng jì shēng* (Herba Taxilli) 15g, *sāng zhī* (Ramulus Mori) 30g, *qín jiāo* (Radix Gentianae Macrophyllae) 15g and *wēi líng xiān* (Radix et Rhizoma Clematidis) 15g to eliminate wind-damp and activate the collaterals. Subtract exterior-relieving medicinals such as *bái zhǐ* (Radix Angelicae Dahuricae) and *niú bàng zǐ* (Fructus Arctii).

Additional Treatment Modalities

1. Chinese Patent Medicine

(1) *Fù Fāng Qīng Dài Wán* (复方青黛丸)

6g, 3 times a day, take the medicine after mixing with boiling water. It functions to clear heat and resolve toxins, invigorate and cool blood, remove ecchymoses, transform stasis and to dispel wind to relieve itching. Suitable for ordinary psoriasis in the active stage.

(2) *Léi Gōng Téng Zhì Jì* (雷公藤制剂)

For *Léi Gōng Téng Piàn* (雷 公 藤 片), 3-4 tablets, 3 times a day; for *Léi Gōng Téng Duō Dài Piàn* (雷公藤多甙片), 2 tablets, 3 times a day. For adults, 40-60mg, take after meals, suitable for all types of psoriasis.

2. Acupuncture and Moxibustion

(1) Acupuncture

【Point Combination】

DU 14	dà zhuī	大椎
BL 13	fèi shù	肺俞
L 11	qū chí	曲池
LI 4	hé gŭ	合谷
SP 10	xuè hăi	血海
SP 6	sān yīn jiāo	三阴交

【Point Modifications】

- For head and face, add GB 20 (*fēng chí*) and LI 20 (*yíng xiāng*).
- For upper limbs, add SJ 6 (*zhī gōu*).
- For lower limbs, add ST 36 and ST 40 (*fēng lóng*).

【Manipulation】

Even reinforcing-reducing method. 10 times as a therapeutic course.

(2) Moxibustion

【Point Selection】

Around affected area.

【Manipulation】

Light a moxa stick and hold 1 cun away from the affected areas to get the sensation of warming and reddening the skin but not painful. 15-20 minutes, 1-2 times a day, 10 days as a course.

(3) Ear Acupuncture Therapy

【Point Selection】

BL 13	fèi shù	肺俞
shenmen	TF4	神门
endocrine	CO18	内分泌

【Point Combination】

heart	CO15	心
large intestine	CO7	大肠

【Manipulation】

Retain the needles for 20-30min, once every other day, 10 days as a course.

(4) Cupping Therapy

【Point Selection】

DU 4	dà zhuī	大椎
DU 13	táo dào	陶道

Bilateral BL 18 (*gān shù*) or BL 20 (*pí shù*).

【Point Combination】

L 11	qū chí	曲池
SP 6	sān yīn jiāo	三阴交

【Manipulation】

(Cupping) Light a cotton stick with 95% alcohol, circle it inside a cup, then place the cup quickly on the selected area, once every other day, 15 times as a course.

3. External Treatments

(1) Wash with a Chinese Herbal Decoction: 30g each of *cè bǎi yè* (Cacumen Platycladi), *chǔ táo yè* (Folium Broussonetiae), *fēng qiú* (Fructus Liquidambaris), *qiān lǐ guāng* (Herba Senecoinis Scandentis), *huáng bǎi*

(Cortex Phellodendri), *dì gǔ pí* (Cortex Lycii), *láng dú* (Radix Euphorbiae Fischerianae) and *bái xiān pí* (Cortex Dictamni). Decoct for a topical wash, once a day.

(2) 5%-10% Sulfur Ointment: Apply on the affected parts, 3 times a day, suitable for stable or dormant phase.

(3) For the active phase (such as agria pattern and erythrodermia pattern), protective agents such as Berberine, *huáng bǎi* (Cortex Phellodendri), and *Qīng Dài Gāo* (青黛膏) or sesame oil are applied on the affected parts, 3 times a day.

4. Simple Prescriptions and Empirical Formulas

(1) *Wáng Shé Jiǔ* (王蛇酒)

Qí shé (Agkistrodon), *jīn mù shé* (Bungarus Fasciatus), *yín hóng shé* (Bungarus Parvus), *yǎn jìng shé* (Cobra) and *wū shāo shē* (Zaocys), soak in wine.

(2) *Tǔ fú líng* (Rhizoma Smilacis Glabrae) 60g, grind into powder and wrap to decoct. Divide in half to take twice. Or use *tǔ fú líng* (Rhizoma Smilacis Glabrae) 60-90g, one dose every day, decoct for oral use.

(3) *Fù Fāng Tǔ Dà Huáng Chá Jì* (复方土大黄搽剂)

20g each of *tǔ dà huáng* (Radix Rumicis Nepalensis), *shé chuáng zǐ* (Fructus Cnidii) and *tǔ jǐn pí* (Cortex Pseudolarix), soak in 1000ml 75% alcohol for 10 days. Filter, add salicylic acid 5g and antipyrine benzoate 12g into the filtrate and mix well. Apply on the affected part twice a day.

(4) *Bá qiā* (Rhizoma Smilacis Chinae) 30-40g a day, soak with 1500 ml warm water for 10 hours, then boil for 40-50 minutes, take after meals 2-3 times a day.

(5) *Huái Huā Fěn* (槐花粉)

Grind *huái huā* (Flos Sophorae) to a powder after stir-frying till yellow. 6g, twice a day, take with warm water after meals, 30 days as a course.

PROGNOSIS

1. Ordinary Psoriasis

If treated properly, this condition can be improved and controlled. But it is still difficult to achieve a complete cure and prevent recurrence. Some patients develop agria psoriasis or erythrodermic psoriasis due to improper medications.

2. Agria Psoriasis, Psoriatic Arthritis and Erythrodermic Psoriasis

These generally have a long course of disease, obstinate and lingering, susceptible to recurrence and with no significant reactions to general treatment. Extensive agria psoriasis is usually complicated by systemic damage such as liver and kidney damage or an unfavorable prognosis due to secondary infections, electrolyte disturbances or depletion. If treated properly some skin damage may occur after healing.

PREVENTIVE HEALTHCARE

Lifestyle Modification

(1) Eat fewer fats and meats. The intake of spicy food and alcohols should be avoided and the intake of fresh fruits and vegetables increased.

(2) Strengthen body constitution and hygiene. Pay attention to avert upper respiratory infections.

(3) Avoid irritating chemicals and pharmaceuticals and the careless use of external medicines. Initially, use mild, non-irritating external medications and then reduce their concentration as the condition improves. The application of strong, external corticosteroid medications over large skin areas on a long-term basis should be avoided.

Dietary Recommendation

People hold various viewpoints about dietary recommendations. Some people advocate a strict avoidance of certain foods while others have no special requirements. The body requires a diverse diet because various nutrients are obtained from different foods. Strict dietetic restraints without a scientific basis not only does little to help recovery but brings more mental pressure to patients. This is not healthy. While blind dietetic restraint is not recommended, patients should pay attention to their daily diet and not eat foods which could aggravate a pathogenic condition. Some suggestions follow:

(1) Eat foods that are low in fat and high in protein. Replace mutton and beef with fish, pork and chicken. Eggs, bean products (tofu) and milk are recommended.

(2) Provide sufficient vitamins and minerals. Eat fresh fruits, vegetables, un-refined grains, beans and cereals. Avoid long cooking time. Dried plum and grapefruit are naturally healthy foods that can help and prevent psoriasis. Both congee soups from *huái huā* (Flos Sophorae) and *líng xiāo huā* (Flos Campsis) and tea have fine preventive and therapeutic effects. It is also beneficial to eat asparagus.

Regulation of Emotional and Mental Health

Because psoriasis creates obstinate skin damage, itching, chronic disease and susceptibility to relapse, it weighs heavy on patients mentally. Thus a skin problem is a disease of both the body and the mind. If the patient is suffering mentally, it is possible for the condition to worsen. If recovery seems unlikely, we should especially put an emphasis on the regulation of emotional and mental health.

Patients should be aware of the features of the disease and not be impatient with the treatments. At the same time, they should try to keep a stable mood and resist negative emotions such as feelings of inferiority and depression. A positive attitude will create a good environment for recuperation.

The patient's family and friends should communicate with them and show compassion for their situation. Doctors also should use suitable treatments for both body and mind and help them resolve their mental suffering.

CLINICAL EXPERIENCES OF RENOWNED PHYSICIANS

Empirical Formulas

1. *Kè Yín Yī Fāng* (克银一方) (Zhu Ren-kang)

【Ingredients】

土茯苓	tŭ fú líng	30g	Rhizoma Smilacis Glabrae
山豆根	shān dòu gēn	10g	Radix et Rhizoma Sophorae Tonkinensis
忍冬藤	rěn dōng téng	15g	Caulis Lonicerae
板蓝根	băn lán gēn	15g	Radix Isatidis
草河车	căo hé chē	15g	Rhizoma Bistortae
白鲜皮	bái xiān pí	15g	Cortex Dictamni
威灵仙	wēi líng xiān	10g	Radix et Rhizoma Clematidis
生甘草	shēng gān căo	6g	Radix et Rhizoma Glycyrrhizae (raw)

【Indications】

Blood heat-wind dryness pattern in the active stage of psoriasis. Flares up rapidly, tiny red dots the size of millet, enlarged or forming plaque, bright red at the base, layers of squamae, easy to exfoliate, punctate hemorrhage (small dots of blood) with redness surrounding it. There is constant new skin damage and isomorphic reaction (localized response to trauma). It is accompanied by irritability and dryness-heat, sore throat and thirst, constipation and brownish urine. There is a red tongue with yellow coating, wiry and rapid pulse or slippery and rapid pulse.

【Modifications】

- For a sore throat and swollen throat, add *jīn yín huā* (Flos Lonicerae), *lián qiào* (Fructus Forsythiae) and *niú bàng zǐ* (Fructus Arctii).
- For cases of thirst add *mài mén dōng* (Raidix Ophiopogonis), *xuán shēn* (Raidix Scrophulariae), *xiān lú gēn* (Fresh Rhizoma Phragmitis) and *xiān máo gēn* (Fresh Rhizoma Imperatae).
- For irritability add *zhī zǐ* (Fructus Gardeniae).
- For dry stool and constipation, add *shēng dà huáng* (raw Radix et Rhizoma Rhei).
- For severe itching add *bái zhǐ* (Radix Angelicae Dahuricae), *bái xiān pí* (Cortex Dictamni) and *bái jí lí* (Fructus Trbuli).
- For dry and thick squamae, add *hǔ zhàng* (Rhizoma et Radix Polygoni Cuspidati).
- For bright red skin damage of large areas, use large dosages of *shēng dì huáng* (Radix Rehmanniae Recens), *mǔ dān pí* (Cortex Moutan) and *chì sháo* (Radix Paeoniae Rubra), add *zǐ cǎo* (Radix Arnebiae).
- For scorching skin damage add *shēng shí gāo* (Gypsum Fivrosum) and *zhī mǔ* (Rhizoma Anemarrhenae).

(Zhu Ren-kang. Clinical Progress of *Kè Yín Fāng* in Treating Psoriasis 克银方治疗银屑病的临床研究进展 . *Journal of Traditional Chinese Medicine* 中医杂志 . 1983, (9): 31)

2. *Kè Yín Èr Fāng* (克银二方) (Zhu Ren-kang)

【Ingredients】

生地黄	shēng dì huáng	30g	Radix Rehmanniae Recens
玄参	xuán shēn	15g	Raidix Scrophulariae
丹参	dān shēn	15g	Radix et Rhizoma Salviae Miltiorrhizae
大青叶	dà qīng yè	15g	Folium Isatidis
白鲜皮	bái xiān pí	15g	Cortex Dictamni

草河车	cǎo hé chē	15g	Rhizoma Bistortae
麻子仁	má zǐ rén	10g	Semen Cannabis
山豆根	shān dòu gēn	10g	Radix et Rhizoma Sophorae Tonkinensis
连翘	lián qiào	10g	Fructus Forsythiae

【Indications】

Blood deficiency and wind dryness psoriasis pattern. Syndrome Characteristics: Usually seen in either the stable or waning stages. The course of the disease is prolonged with erythema from a coin size to large sizes. Dry skin, pink plaque, dry with layers and layers of scales that easily fall off when touched. Or there may be very chapped skin with bleeding that is itchy or painful. Clear lightly coated tongue and a wiry and thready pulse.

【Modifications】

➢ For thirst add *tiān mén dōng* (Radix Asparagi), *mài mén dōng* (Raidix Ophiopogonis) and *tiān huā fěn* (Radix Trichosanthis).

➢ For constipation add *hé shǒu wū* (Radix Polygoni Multiflori), *dāng guī* (Radix Angelicae Sinensis) and *ròu cóng róng* (Herba Cistanches).

➢ For itching add *bái xiān pí* (Cortex Dictamni) and *bái zhǐ* (Radix Angelicae Dahuricae).

➢ For dark red skin damage add *dāng guī wěi* (End of Radix Angelicae Sinensis), *táo rén* (Semen Persicae) and *hóng huā* (Flos Carthami).

➢ For thick and hardened skin damage, add *sān léng* (Rhizoma Sparganii) and *é zhú* (Rhizoma Curcumae).

➢ For dry and chapped skin damage, add *běi shā shēn* (Radix Glehniae) and *mài mén dōng* (Raidix Ophiopogonis).

➢ For thick scaling add *dāng guī* (Radix Angelicae Sinensis) and *jī xuè téng* (Caulis Spatholobi).

(Zhu Ren-kang. Clinical Progress of *Kè Yín Fāng* in Treating Psoriasis

克银方治疗银屑病的临床研究进展 . *Journal of Traditional Chinese Medicine* 中医杂志 . 1983, (9): 31)

3. *Bái Gē Yī Hào* (白疙一号) (Zhang Zhi-li)

【Ingredients】

紫草根	zǐ cǎo gēn	15g	Radix Arnebiae
茜草根	qiàn cǎo gēn	15g	Radix et Rhizoma Rubiae
大青叶	dà qīng yè	30g	Folium Isatidis
白茅根	bái máo gēn	30g	Rhizoma Imperatae
槐花	huái huā	30g	Flos Sophorae
山豆根	shān dòu gēn	6g	Radix et Rhizoma Sophorae Tonkinensis
生地	shēng dì huáng	30g	Radix Rehmanniae Recens
丹皮	dān pí	15g	Cortex Moutan
丹参	dān shēn	15g	Radix et Rhizoma Salviae Miltiorrhizae
赤芍	chì sháo	15g	Radix Paeoniae Rubra

【Indications】

Psoriasis of the blood heat pattern in the active phase. Syndrome characteristics: The rapid and consistent growth of new erythema prevents new scales from covering it. It is usually accompanied by agitation and the propensity to anger. Dry mouth and throat, dry stool and constipation, scanty brownish urine. Red tongue with a thin white or yellow coating, wiry and slippery or rapid pulse.

【Modifications】

➢ For pathological changes concentrated in the lower part of body, add *quán guā lóu* (Fructus et Semen Trichosanthis), use large dosages of *bǎn lán gēn* (Radix Isatidis).

➢ For severe wind-pruritus add *bái xiān pí* (Cortex Dictamni) and *cì jí lí* (Fructus Trbuli).

➢ For cases of pathogenic damp with a light tongue body and white greasy coating, conspicuous skin damage, add *shēng yǐ rén* (raw Semen Coicis), *fáng jǐ* (Radix Stephaniae Tetrandrae) and *yīn chén* (Herba

Artemisiae Scopariae).

➢ For dry stool add *dà huáng* (Radix et Rhizoma Rhei) and *zhī zǐ* (raw Fructus Gardeniae).

➢ For strong heat add *lóng dǎn cǎo* (Radix Gentianae) and *huáng qín* (Radix Scutellariae).

➢ For cases with pharyngitis and tonsillitis, add *jīn yín huā* (Flos Lonicerae), *lián qiào* (Fructus Forsythiae) and *jǐn dēng lóng* (Calyx seu fructus Physalis).

(Wang Ping, et al. Treatment and Clinical Study of Psoriasis of Zhang Zhi-li by Syndrome Differentiation (One) 张志礼中医辨证治疗银屑病方法及临床研究(一). *Chinese Journal of Dermatovenereology of Integrated Traditional and Western Medicine* 中国中西医结合皮肤性病学杂志. 2004, 3(4): 191-193.)

4. *Bái Gē Èr Hào* (白疙二号) (Zhang Zhi-li)

【Ingredients】

当归	dāng guī	10g	Radix Angelicae Sinensis
鸡血藤	jī xuè téng	30g	Caulis Spatholobi
丹参	dān shēn	15g	Radix et Rhizoma Salviae Miltiorrhizae
天门冬	tiān mén dōng	10g	Radix Asparagi
麦门冬	mài mén dōng	10g	Raidix Ophiopogonis
生地	shēng dì huáng	30g	Radix Rehmanniae Recens
土茯苓	tǔ fú líng	30g	Rhizoma Smilacis Glabrae
白术	bái zhú	10g	Fructus Aurantii
枳壳	zhǐ qiào	10g	Fructus Forsythiae
薏米	yì mǐ	30g	Semen Coicis

【Indications】

Psoriasis of wind-heat and blood dryness pattern in a stable phase. Here the pathogenic condition is relatively stable but chronic. The color of the lesions is becoming lighter and with few new skin erythema. The original erythema is fading away. Some have the size and appearance of a coin or else they are grouped together with a few superficial squamae, adhering closely. There are few general symptoms. The tongue is light red or a red tongue tip with a light tongue body with a scanty coating. The pulse is moderate or deep and thready.

【Modifications】

- For Spleen deficiency with damp add *yì yǐ rén* (raw Semen Coicis), *bái zhú* (Rhizoma Atractylodis Macrocephalae), *fú líng* (Poria) and *bái biǎn dòu* (Semen Lablab Album).
- For severe wind-pruritus add *cì jí lí* (Fructus Trbuli) and *kǔ shēn* (Radix Sophorae Flavescentis).
- For yin deficiency and blood heat, red tongue with a scanty coating, add *xuán shēn* (Raidix Scrophulariae), *dì gǔ pí* (Cortex Lycii) and *dān pí* (Cortex Moutan).

(Wang Ping, et al. Treatment and Clinical Study of Psoriasis of Zhang Zhi-li by Syndrome Differentiation (One) 张志礼中医辨证治疗银屑病方法及临床研究 (一). *Chinese Journal of Dermatovenereology of Integrated Traditional and Western Medicine* 中国中西医结合皮肤性病学杂志. 2004, 3(4): 191-193.)

5. *Bái Gē Sān Hào* (白疕三号) (Zhang Zhi-li)

【Ingredients】

桃仁	táo rén	15g	Semen Persicae
红花	hóng huā	15g	Flos Carthami
三棱	sān léng	15g	Rhizoma Sparganii
莪术	é zhú	15g	Rhizoma Curcumae
丹参	dān shēn	15g	Radix et Rhizoma Salviae Miltiorrhizae
鸡血藤	jī xuè téng	30g	Caulis Spatholobi
鬼箭羽	guǐ jiàn yǔ	30g	Lignum Suberalatum Evonymi
陈皮	chén pí	10g	Pericarpium Citri Reticulatae
白花蛇舌草	bái huā shé shé cǎo	30g	Herba Hedyotis
土茯苓	tǔ fú líng	30g	Rhizoma Smilacis Glabrae

薏米	yì mǐ	30g	Semen Coicis
重楼	chóng lóu	15g	Rhzoma Bistortae

【Indications】

Psoriasis with a blood stasis pattern in the stable phase. Patients are often older in age with a prolonged and long history of the disease. The skin damage is like leather with thick scales and severe itching. Dark purple tongue or stasis spots and maculae. The pulse is rough or deep and moderate.

【Modifications】

➢ For scanty menstrual blood or with blood clots, add *yì mǔ cǎo* (Herba Leonuri) and *dāng guī* (Radix Angelicae Sinensis). When complicated by Liver constraint and qi stagnation, add *chái hú* (Radix Bupleuri), *zhǐ qiào* (Fructus Aurantii) and *xiāng fù* (Rhizoma Cyperi).

➢ For disharmony of yin and yang add *shǒu wū téng* (Caulis Polygoni Multiflori) and *gōu téng* (Ramulus Uncariae Cum Uncis).

➢ For scorching skin damage add *shēng shí gāo* (Gypsum Fivrosum) and *zhī mǔ* (Rhizoma Anemarrhenae).

(Wang Ping, et al. Treatment and Clinical Study of Psoriasis of Zhang Zhi-li by Syndrome Differentiation (One) 张志礼中医辨证治疗银屑病方法及临床研究(一). *Chinese Journal of Dermatovenereology of Integrated Traditional and Western Medicine* 中国中西医结合皮肤性病学杂志. 2004, 3(4): 191-193.)

Selected Case Studies

1. Case Studies of Zhu Ren-kang

(1) Wind-heat Stagnation, Damaging Yin and Transforming into Dryness

【Initial Visit】

Mr Xu, age 40. Initial visit time: May 26th 1980.

A half year ago, an initial itchy rash appeared on the back of the hand and then gradually extended over the entire body. After the application of Chlorphenamine Maleate, vitamin C and hydrocortisone, the condition was controlled a little. Around January, from the original focal point of infection, erythema and blisters (vesicopustule) developed and got worse day by day.

Examination: The back of the hand and trunk have erythema lesions of unequal size. Some of the papules appear to be filled with liquid and have effusion (oozing) and there is some erosion of the areas. The tongue is enlarged and slightly red with a thin yellow coating. The pulse is soggy and rapid.

【Pattern Differentiation】

Wind-heat accumulation, consumed yin and transformed into dryness.

【Treatment Principle】

Cool blood and clear heat, tonify yin to moisten dryness.

【Prescription】

生地黄	shēng dì huáng	30g	Radix Rehmanniae Recens
生槐花	shēng huái huā	30g	Flos Sophorae (raw)
紫草	zǐ cǎo	15g	Radix Arnebiae
牡丹皮	mǔ dān pí	9g	Cortex Moutan
赤芍	chì sháo	9g	Radix Paeoniae Rubra
麻仁	má rén	15g	Semen Cannabis
枳壳	zhǐ qiào	9g	Fructus Aurantii
麦门冬	mài mén dōng	9g	Raidix Ophiopogonis
大青叶	dà qīng yè	9g	Folium Isatidis

Decoct in water, one dose a day, take ten doses and use *Hóng Yóu Gāo* (红油膏) externally, once a day.

【Second Visit】

After medication, the skin damage gradually subsided in the leg and on the other parts in an obvious reduction in scaling. The patient continued to take the former prescription with the dosages of *huǒ má rén*

(Semen Cannabis) changed to 9g and *dà qīng yè* (Folium Isatidis) to 15g for 10 doses.

【Third Visit】

Skin damage in the trunk and upper limbs have subsided. After subsiding on the lower limbs, new eruptions appeared. Dry mouth and thirst, thin yellow tongue coating. The former formula was again used with *huáng qín* (Radix Scutellariae) 9g and *tiān huā fěn* (Radix Trichosanthis) 9g added. 10 doses were given to consolidate the therapeutic effect.

(Edited by Guang An Men Hospital of Academy Institute of Chinese Medicine. *Clinical Experience Collection of Zhu Ren-kang* 朱仁康临床经验集. People's Medical Publishing House 人民卫生出版社, 1979: 152)

(2) Blood-heat and Wind Dryness

【Initial Visit】

Male, age 10. Initial visit time: May 24th, 1985.

Five years ago, the four limbs and trunk developed flaky skin and psoriasis. There was underlying redness, flaking of skin-exfoliation, itching. It was gradually spreading all over the body along with running sores. The pathogenic conditions were not improved after treatment at a major hospital. Taking dextrosulfenidol once, proved effective for a short time, but then erupted soon after on the entire body.

Examination: Except for the face there was whole body redness (erubescence), scaling, running sores which was especially severe on the chest, back and limbs. This was accompanied by nausea and poor appetite. When the skin damage developed, the appetite improved but when the skin got better the appetite got worse. Red and crimson tongue, peeled coating, thready and rapid pulse.

【Pattern Differentiation】

Blood heat and wind dryness consumed yin, strong heat transformed into toxicity.

【Treatment Principle】

Cool blood, clear heat and resolve toxins, tonify yin and moisten dryness.

【Prescription】

生地	shēng dì huáng	30g	Radix Rehmanniae Recens
丹参	dān shēn	15g	Radix et Rhizoma Salviae Miltiorrhizae
玄参	xuán shēn	10g	Raidix Scrophulariae
连翘	lián qiào	10g	Fructus Forsythiae
石斛	shí hú	10g	Herba Dendrobii
银花	jīn yín huā	10g	Flos Lonicerae
麦冬	mài dōng	10g	Raidix Ophiopogonis
生甘草	shēng gān cǎo	6g	Radix et Rhizoma Glycyrrhizae (raw)

Decoct in water, one dose a day, 10 doses.

【Second Visit】

Red flushing relieved after medication, pustula dried and less crusted. Using the last formula and *tiān huā fěn* (Radix Trichosanthis) 10g and *bái máo gēn* (Rhizoma Imperatae) 10g were added. Took 7 doses.

【Third Visit】

Most parts of the skin damage subsided. Relapse after withdrawal of the herbs for one week, with flushing and pustules in the chest and back. Poor appetite.

【Prescription】

生地	shēng dì	30g	Radix Rehmanniae Recens
鸡内金	jī nèi jīn	10g	Endothelium Corneum Gigeriae Galli
连翘	lián qiào	10g	Fructus Forsythiae
石斛	shí hú	10g	Herba Dendrobii
银花	jīn yín huā	10g	Flos Lonicerae
麦冬	mài dōng	10g	Raidix Ophiopogonis
丹皮	dān pí	10g	Cortex Moutan
赤勺	chì sháo	10g	Radix Paeoniae Rubra

7 doses.

【Fourth Visit】

After medication, redness and pustules on the chest and back diminished with a few pustules appeared on the right lower limb. Red crimson tongue, slightly peeled coating. Referring to the above formula, *shēng gǔ yá* (Fructus Setariae Germinatus) 10g was added, 7 doses.

【Fifth Visit】

After taking the herbs, the pustules in the right lower limb formed a scab and then fell off. There was slight exfoliation and a good appetite. The tongue and pulse were the same as the fourth visit. Fourth visit formula, took 7 doses.

【Sixth Visit】

Mostly receded, generally no new pustules, dark red in the areas of skin damage, few scales, poor appetite again, took the third visit formula and added *huò xiāng* (Herba Pogostemonis) 8g, 14 doses.

【Seventh Visit】

Skin damage generally gone, smooth skin, remaining hyperpigmentation, appetite improved. From the sixth formula subtracted *huò xiāng* (Herba Pogostemonis), took 7 doses. Completely cured.

(Pang Jian-zhong. *Selected Comments on Ancient and Modern Case Studies* 中医古今医案精髓选评 . Beijing: College Publishing House 学苑出版社 , 1998: 2478-2479.)

2. Case Studies of Zhang Zhi-li

Blood Stasis

【Initial Visit】

Female, age 49, initial visit time: July 22nd 1999.

Eighteen years ago, rash occurred on the head, covered with dry silvery scaling, diagnosed as psoriasis. No improvement was seen after treatment, and the erythema gradually increased over the entire body with itching.

Examination: Argentate (silver-white) scaling on the head, fleshy plaque in chest, back and thighs, dark red in color. Dark purple tongue, white coating, deep and moderate pulse.

【Pattern Differentiation】

Blood stasis.

【Treatment Principle】

Invigorate blood to remove stasis, eliminate dampness and resolve toxins.

【Prescription】

桃仁	táo rén	10g	Semen Persicae
红花	hóng huā	10g	Flos Carthami
茜草	qiàn cǎo	15g	Radix et Rhizoma Rubiae
板蓝根	bǎn lán gēn	30g	Radix Isatidis
三棱	sān léng	10g	Rhizoma Sparganii
莪术	é zhú	10g	Rhizoma Curcumae
大青叶	dà qīng yè	30g	Folium Isatidis
紫草	zǐ cǎo	15g	Radix Paeoniae Rubra
生槐花	shēng huái huā	30g	Flos Sophorae (raw)
土茯苓	tǔ fú líng	30g	Rhizoma Smilacis Glabrae
白鲜皮	bái xiān pí	30g	Cortex Dictamni
苦参	kǔ shēn	15g	Radix Sophorae Flavescentis
生地黄	shēng dì huáng	15g	Radix Rehmanniae Recens

Decoct in water, one dose a day. 28 doses.

5% unguentum acidi salicylici for external use.

【Second Visit】

After medication, the skin damage was relatively decreased from before, fleshy sections seemed to rise up from under the skin and the scales were relatively fewer. Using the last formula, added *yì yǐ rén* (Semen Coicis) 30g and *zhǐ qiào* (Fructus Aurantii) 10g, took 28 doses.

【Third Visit】

Skin damage generally receded, macules of hyperpigmentation due to inflammation remained, continued to take the second visit formula to strengthen the treatment.

(Zhang Zhi-li. *Zhang Zhi-li's Important Clinical Experience of Dermatonosis* 张志礼皮肤病临床经验辑要 .The Medicine Science and Technology Press of China 中国医药科技出版社 , 2001: 266-267.)

3. Case Studies of Zhao Bing-nan

Damp-heat Accumulation, Blood-heat Hyperactivity-blazing.

【Initial Visit】

Male, age 30. Initial visit time: July 1st 1964.

Skin rash on the four limbs for over three years, occurred every winter and spring with remission in the summer and autumn. He was diagnosed with psoriasis and treated many times. In May of this year, gradually the whole body became red with white scales at the surface and with diffused red swelling of the lower limbs. There was dry stool and brownish urine.

Examination: Erythema and white squamae (scales) on the scalp; scattered coin sized scaly erythema on the lower abdomen, waist and buttocks, erythema surrounding elbow and knee joints, warmth in the lower limbs and with tiny squamae. Extensive keratinization and desquamation on the soles of the feet and palms of the hand. Red tongue body and white coating, rapid pulse .

【Pattern Differentiation】

Accumulated damp-heat, blood-heat hyperactivity-blazing.

【Treatment Principle】

Clear heat and remove dampness, cool blood and invigorate blood.

【Prescription】

藏红花	zàng hóng huā	4.5g	Stigma Croci
黄柏	huáng bǎi	9g	Cortex Phellodendri
生栀子	shēng zhī zǐ	9g	Fructus Gardeniae（raw）
牡丹皮	mǔ dān pí	9g	Cortex Moutan

泽泻	zé xiè	9g	Rhizoma Alismatis
生槐花	huái huā	30g	Flos Sophorae (raw)
黄芩	huáng qín	9g	Radix Scutellariae
陈蒿	yīn chén hāo	9g	Herba Artemisiae Scopariae
车前子	chē qián zĭ	9g	Semen Plantaginis
生地	shēng dì huáng	30g	Radix Rehmanniae Recens
红条紫草	zĭ căo	9g	Radix Arnebiae
凌霄花	líng xiāo huā	9g	Flos Campsis
土茯苓	tŭ fú líng	9g	Rhizoma Smilacis Glabrae
甘草	gān căo	15g	Radix et Rhizoma Glycyrrhizae

Decoct in water, one dose a day. Three doses.

Pŭ Lián Ruăn Gāo (普连软膏) for external use.

【Second Visit】

Skin redness turned darker after medication, small patches of healthy skin appeared in the reddened regions, and the damaged areas were differentiated, itching. To the above formula took out *mŭ dān pí* (Cortex Moutan), added *bái xiān pí* (Cortex Dictamni) and *dà huáng* (Radix et Rhizoma Rhei). Took three doses.

【Third Visit】

Skin redness was lighter than that of the second visit. The red skin of the leg calf has obviously cleared up with reduced itching. Referring to the formula of the initial visit, added *mù tōng* (Caulis Clematis Armandii), took 3 doses.

【Fourth Visit】

Skin redness generally gone after taking the medication, original psoriasis vulgaris damage remained. Referring to the formula of the third visit, subtract *xī hóng huā* (Stigma Croci) and added *shú dì huáng* (Radix Rehmanniae Praeparata), took 3 doses.

【Fifth Visit】

The herb formula took away much of the damage with only a few remaining red spots. Keratinization on the palms and soles was better than before. Lighter tongue body, submerged and relaxed pulse. The treatment principle was to remove dampness and enrich the blood to moisten the skin.

【Prescription】

生地	shēng dì huáng	30g	Radix Rehmanniae Recens
熟地	shú dì huáng	15g	Radix Rehmanniae Praeparata
炒黄柏	chǎo huáng bǎi	9g	Parched Cortex Phellodendri Tostum
生栀子	shēng zhī zǐ	9g	Fructus Gardeniae (raw)
泽泻	zé xiè	9g	Rhizoma Alismatis
白鲜皮	bái xiān pí	30g	Cortex Dictamni
当归	dāng guī	9g	Radix Angelicae Sinensis
土茯苓	tǔ fú líng	30g	Rhizoma Smilacis Glabrae
车前子	chē qián zǐ	9g	Semen Plantaginis
木通	mù tōng	6g	Caulis Clematis Armandii
生槐花	shēng huái huā	30g	Flos Sophorae (raw)
甘草	gān cǎo	6g	Radix et Rhizoma Glycyrrhizae

After successive 15 doses, the patient was clinically healed.

(Beijing College of Chinese Medicine, *Clinical Experience Collection of Zhao Bing-nan* 赵炳南临床经验集 . Beijing: People's Medical Publishing House 人民卫生出版社 , 1975: 224-225)

Discussions

1. Zhu Ren-kang's Comments on Psoriasis

In Chinese medicine, psoriasis is listed as wind or *Xuan* (often translated as tinea) and *Bai Bi Feng* (white dagger wind). Because of its distinct skin damage and layers of squamae, it is also known as *Song Pi Xie* (pine tree bark) and *Bai Ke Bing* (white shell illness).

The major cause is blood-heat. With blood-heat constitution, exopathogenic/external wind invades the body, then blood-heat generates wind, and wind dryness causes reddening, desquamation (flaky skin), and the consumption of yin and blood. This finally results in yin deficiency and blood dryness which fails to nourish the skin. Because of this, dry skin and layers of white scales appear.

(1) Blood-heat

It is often seen in the active stage of psoriasis. It is caused by internal excessive blood-heat with exogenous wind-evil attacking, impairing *ying*-blood and transforming to dryness.

It manifests as bright red skin damage which develops quickly, with constant new skin damage, irritability, thirst, dry stool. Red and purple tongue, yellow coating, wiry and slippery pulse.

The treatment principle is to cool blood, clear heat and resolve toxins.

The formula is *Tǔ Fú Líng Tāng* (土茯苓汤).

生地	shēng dì huáng	30g	Radix Rehmanniae Recens
紫草	zǐ cǎo	15g	Radix Arnebiae
生槐花	shēng huái huā	30g	Flos Sophorae (raw)
土茯苓	tǔ fú líng	30g	Rhizoma Smilacis Glabrae
蚤休	zǎo xiū	15g	Rhzoma Bistortae
白鲜皮	bái xiān pí	15g	Cortex Dictamni
大青叶	dà qīng yè	15g	Folium Isatidis
山豆根	shān dòu gēn	9g	Radix et Rhizoma Sophorae Tonkinensis
忍冬藤	rěn dōng téng	15g	Caulis Lonicerae
生甘草	gān cǎo	6g	Radix et Rhizoma Glycyrrhizae (raw)

(2) Blood Dryness

It is often seen in the stable stage of psoriasis.

With weak body constitution, insufficient blood and qi or chronic wind dryness impair yin and blood; deficient blood generates wind and transforms into dryness failing to nourish the skin. Dry skin, erythroic plaque, layers of squamae, constant new erythema. Light tongue, clear coating, wiry and thready pulse.

Treatment principle is primarily enriching and invigorating blood, tonifying yin to moisten dryness.

生地黄	shēng dì huáng	15g	Radix Rehmanniae Recens
熟地黄	shú dì huáng	15g	Radix Rehmanniae Praeparata
当归	dāng guī	12g	Radix Angelicae Sinensis
桃仁	táo rén	9g	Semen Persicae
红花	hóng huā	9g	Flos Carthami
玄参	xuán shēn	9g	Raidix Scrophulariae
天门冬	tiān mén dōng	9g	Radix Asparagi
麦门冬	mài mén dōng	9g	Raidix Ophiopogonis
麻子仁	má zǐ rén	9g	Semen Cannabis
甘草	gān cǎo	6g	Radix et Rhizoma Glycyrrhizae

(3) Wind-damp

It is caused by pathogenic wind-damp entering the collaterals, consuming nutritive blood and transforming to dryness.

It manifests as general skin damage all over the body, aching joints, deformation and abnormalities in the finger joints that are unable to straighten. Thin, white, greasy tongue fur, wiry and slippery pulse.

The treatment principle is to activate the collaterals to invigorate blood, expel wind and eliminate dampness.

桂枝	guì zhī	9g	Ramulus Cinnamomi
当归	dāng guī	12g	Radix Angelicae Sinensis
赤芍	chì sháo	12g	Radix Paeoniae Rubra
知母	zhī mǔ	9g	Rhizoma Anemarrhenae
桑寄生	sāng jì shēng	9g	Herba Taxilli
防风	fáng fēng	9g	Radix Saposhnikoviae
桑枝	sāng zhī	15g	Ramulus Mori
怀牛膝	huái niú xī	9g	Radix Acanthopanacis Bidentatae
忍冬藤	rěn dōng téng	9g	Caulis Lonicerae
鸡血藤	jī xuè téng	30g	Caulis Spatholobi
甘草	gān cǎo	6g	Radix et Rhizoma Glycyrrhizae

(4) Toxic Heat

It is caused by pathogenic wind, damp and heat accumulating for a long period and transforming to toxicity.

It manifests as skin damage, pustules in the deep skin of both palms, red tongue, thin yellow coating, wiry slippery and rapid pulse.

The treatment principle is aimed at eliminating dampness and clearing heat, removing wind and resolving toxins.

乌梢蛇	wū shāo shé	9g	Zaocys
秦艽	qín jiāo	9g	Radix Gentianae Macrophyllae
漏芦	lòu lú	9g	Radix Rhapontici
大黄	dà huáng	6g	Radix et Rhizoma Rhei
黄连	huáng lián	9g	Rhizoma Coptidis
防风	fáng fēng	6g	Radix Saposhnikoviae
生槐花	shēng huái huā	9g	Flos Sophorae (raw)
土茯苓	tǔ fú líng	30g	Rhizoma Smilacis Glabrae
苦参	kǔ shēn	9g	Radix Sophorae Flavescentis
苍术	cāng zhú	9g	Rhizoma Atractylodis
白术	bái zhú	9g	Rhizoma Atractylodis Macrocephala
白鲜皮	bái xiān pí	9g	Cortex Dictamni

External Treatment

1) For skin damage in the acute stage, prescribe *Yù Huáng Gāo* (玉黄膏) 30g, and add 9g of *huáng bǎi* powder (Cortex Phellodendri), 1-2 times a day.

2) For skin damage in the stable stage, apply *Hóng Fěn Gāo* (红粉膏) and *Hóng Yóu Gāo* (红油膏), once a day. Attention: Choose a small area of skin for a dermal test when applying the ointment for the first time. If there are no hypersensitive reactions then apply it on the other parts of the skin. Observe the skin changes during usage and be careful when applying to large areas of skin damage.

(Zhu Ren-kang. *Clinical Experience Collection of Zhu Ren-kang* 朱仁康临床经验集 . Beijing: People's Medical Publishing House 人民卫生出版社 , 1979: 155)

2. Ou-yang Heng's Comments on Generalized Pustule Type of Psoriasis

Generalized pustule pattern is a serious condition of psoriasis. These cases are rare in the clinical with an extremely high death rate. Doctors are often frustrated about how to treat these patients. We have now accumulated some experiences through many years of treating the disease. They are elaborated as follows:

(1) It is crucial with high fever to differentiate according to the warm disease

The correct differentiation of complicated syndromes and signs most directly influences therapeutic efficacy. One should focus close attention to fevers in the clinic. Look at the basis of the disease and correlate them to the basic rules of febrile diseases. Apply warm disease differentiation to firmly establish the treatment principles. Apply them to make a comprehensive analysis which is based on the progression of the disease in the body. Do not confine your diagnosis to the local skin damage. Fever is not only a major symptom, but also the important turning point of the disease. Because skin damage is related to heat, the retreating of heat results in a decrease of the pustules. But with the relapse of heat, then the disease is worsening. The differentiation of the syndrome should be the guideline to establish the treatment.

(2) The interplay between healthy energy and pathogens can be divided into three stages

a. **High fever is a critically dangerous time for the patient.** There can be a unremitting high fever, usually between 40-42℃ (104-108 F), generalized erythema, dense pustules, ragged with erosion, effusion and incrustation. It can be accompanied by general symptoms of drowsiness, irritation-vexation, thirst, constipation, toxic urine, a crimson tongue, thick yellow coating or with yellow prickles, and a wiry and rapid pulse.

The syndromes are heat entering the qi and nutritive level, intense heat toxins blazing, flourishing pathogens and strong right qi. The treatment principle is to clear heat to purge fire. Use the formula *Liáng Xuè Jiě Dú Tāng* (凉血解毒汤), and add *qīng dài* (Indigo Naturalis), *zǐ cǎo* (Radix Arnebiae) and *láng dú* (Radix Euphorbiae Fischerianae). If necessary, combine this with other medicinals for strengthening the body resistance and protecting yin such as *xī yáng shēn* (Radix Panacis Quinque folii) and *xuán shēn* (Raidix Scrophulariae).

b. **When the fever recedes**: When proper treatment is prescribed during the high fever stage, then it enters into this stage. The body temperature goes below 39℃, erythema and pustules have stopped developing but there is mental tiredness, poor appetite, dry mouth, thirst but with no desire to drink, red tongue with scanty coating, thready and rapid pulse. The patterns are intense heat toxicity consuming qi and yin, pathogens flourishing and a deficiency of upright (*zheng*) qi. The treatment principle is primarily resolving toxins, benefiting qi and enriching yin. The formulas are *Zhú Yè Shí Gāo Tāng* (竹叶石膏汤) and *Huáng Lián Jiě Dú Tāng* (黄连解毒汤) and modified *Jū Tōng Yù Nǚ Jiān* (鞠通玉女煎).

c. **Stable convalescence stage**: Manifests as a normal body temperature, decreased skin damage, general desquamation (flaking), extreme exhaustion, poor appetite, dry mouth and lips, peeled tongue, flushed face, scanty or no coating on the tongue, weak, thready and rapid pulse. The treatment principle is to enrich Stomach yin and the formulas are *Yì Wèi Tāng* (益胃汤), *Zēng Yè Tāng* (增液汤) adding *xī yáng shēn* (Radix Panacis Quinquefolii).

(3) It is best to apply a combination of treatments for complicated and dangerous pathogenic conditions

a. One should give priority to heat conditions because the clinical condition of fever is complex and changeable. Therefore one cannot always just follow the three causative factors of fever: internal factors, medication and common cold or secondary infections. Corresponding strategies should be used according to the different causative factors.

b. **Deal with skin damage properly**: Improper treatment of skin damage often results in secondary infections which aggravates the pathogenic conditions. So it is important to treat skin damage properly. Methods: Apply *Pí Sǔn Yī Hào* (皮损 1 号) for an external wash. It consists of *sāng bái pí* (Cortex Mori), *dì gǔ pí* (Cortex Lycii), *bái xiān pí* (Cortex Dictamni), *máng xiāo* (Natrii Sulfas), *huáng bǎi* (Cortex Phellodendri), *huáng lián* (Rhizoma Coptidis), *dà qīng yè* (Folium Isatidis) and *lòu lú* (Radix Rhapontici). Or treat skin damaged areas topically with *qīng dài* (Indigo Naturalis) in teel oil. In the later stage, apply *Yào Xūn Yī Hào* (药熏 I 号). For a medicated or steam bath, use *kǔ shēn* (Radix Sophorae Flavescentis), *shé chuáng zǐ* (Fructus Cnidii), *bái xiān pí* (Cortex Dictamni), *bái sháo* (Raidix Paeoniae Alba) and *zǐ sū* (Folium Perilae) achieving good results. Choose different herbs according to the skin damage: for generalized erythema like erythroderma, use *Jīng Wàn Hóng Tàng Shāng Gāo* (京万红烫伤膏) externally. For dry skin and large amount of scales (squamae) use *Qīng Dài Gāo* (青黛膏) externally. For erosion skin damage, apply *Liù Yī Sǎn* (六一散) externally. When the pathogenic conditions are controlled and transform to an ordinary pattern, use an appropriate Chinese medicated bath.

c. **Make note of consolidating qi and yin**: High fever can easily consume yin and fluids. Patients have differing degrees of redness on their lips, dry mouth and thirst, red peeled tongue, and thready pulse. The condition of Stomach qi and yin determines the prognosis of the disease. Therefore the method of benefiting qi and enriching yin should be continued throughout the whole therapy (but should be prescribed cautiously in patients with yin and fluid deficiency). Meanwhile, adequate therapy courses are recommended to be taken. Prescribe biomedicine rationally, and augment with nursing care. Maintaining a peaceful environment and sanitary conditions should not be ignored.

3. Zhou Ming-qi's Comments on Psoriasis

(1) Establish Principles Based on Etiology and the Relevance to Blood-heat, Dryness and Stasis

Zhou believes the primary cause of psoriasis is blood heat, which manifests as wind, dryness and stasis. Although psoriasis is also caused by invasion from the six pathogenic factors, the majority of the time it is the result of blood-heat generating wind. This wind engenders dryness. Consequently the root of the syndrome always belongs to a yang, heat and excess pattern, and the pathogenesis is heat retention in the blood of the collaterals. Many times psoriasis is caused by internal causes, as well as by a pathogenic combination of internal and external factors that can be aggravated by external pathogens. Macula eruption of psoriasis is caused by blood-heat retention spreading to the vessels and collaterals. This abundance of heat creates the red spots on the exterior skin. Excessive heat generates wind causing dryness. Scales then emerge and transform into dryness due to skin malnutrition, consuming yin over time. This in turn aggravates dryness and heat syndromes. When the skin fails to be nourished, then layers of squamae appear. The main treatment principle is to clear heat and cool blood, as well as eliminate wind, resolve toxins and tonify yin to moisten dryness.

(2) Two Types and Four Differentiations

Two types diagnosis means that psoriasis is either an excess wind-blood-heat pattern or a wind-heat-blood dryness pattern. The former is the active stage of psoriasis, and the latter is its stable stage.

The four differentiations are:

1) Differentiate and prioritize the root cause and the symptoms: Find the central issues between the root and branch and treat the transformations between blood-heat engendering wind, dryness and stasis.

2) Differentiation between excess and deficiency: Consider the constitution, the condition of healthy qi and pathogens and the length of the disease time and age.

3) Differentiation of macula eruption: Extensive red macular eruptions can gradually form generalized scaling that easily exfoliates. The main cause of bleeding after exfoliation or constant macula eruption is excessive wind and toxic heat in the blood. This creates dark or light red erythema and thick layers of dry squamae that are not easily dislodged. When there is little susceptibility to bleeding after exfoliation (or no new erythema) this is primarily caused by blood dryness and blood stasis failing to nourish the skin.

4) Differentiation of complicated syndromes: Due to different body constitutions and pathogens, psoriasis is often complicated by simultaneous conditions of dampness, stasis and deficiency. Some of these are primary causes and some are secondary conditions. Differentiating the innumerable variations of the syndrome can only enhance the therapeutic effects.

PERSPECTIVES OF INTEGRATIVE MEDICINE

Challenges and Solutions

Psoriasis is an obstinate and recurrent dermatologic disease which brings patients great physical and psychological suffering. Research has been extensive in recent years, but there still have been no significant breakthroughs.

Challenge #1: Etiology Aspects

There are many factors that cause psoriasis. These include heredity, infections, spirit-mind issues and endocrine, metabolic and immunologic disorders. So far, no definitive mechanisms of the illness have been determined.

Challenge #2: Treatment Aspects

Psoriasis treatment is a problem that many around the world have researched. Practitioners of biomedicine prescribe antitumor drugs, immune depressants, corticosteroid hormones, antibiotics and vitamins. Some work well but also have such strong side effects that they are limited in their application. Chinese medicine treats the root of the disease by combining syndrome differentiation while considering the typing and staging. Clinically, a number of empirical and modified formulas have very good and proven therapeutic effects but progress may be slow. Most patients get relief from treatment but few are completely cured. Both biomedicine and Chinese medicine lack the specific medicines of a definitive treatment or cure.

Challenge #3: Problem of Recurrence

The recurrence of psoriasis has long been a problem for both doctors and patients. At present, no drug can prevent relapse. This presents a difficulty because it creates a loss of confidence in the therapeutic treatment.

Solutions

Based on the above problems, we should do research in several directions:

1) Do further research into the etiology and mechanisms of psoriasis. Only through the fundamental understanding of the mechanisms will therapeutic and preventative breakthroughs be found.

2) Apply integrative medicine and manufacture safe and effective

drugs. Accent the positives of the quick efficacy of biomedicine with the advantages of the safety and relatively fewer side effects of Chinese medicine. Meanwhile, do studies on empirical and modified formulas to get a better understanding of their exact therapeutic effects to get a better understanding of their mechanisms of action.

3) Conduct preventative and therapeutic education with a modern medical point of view, considering biological, psychological and social factors holistically. Emphasize psychological regulation in treatment and treat patients with caring and understanding.

Empirical studies have shown that psoriasis patients have abnormal laboratory examinations even after healing from psoriasis clinically. Actual lab reports are unusual in that the immune markers remain within the epidermis. Microcirculation at the healed areas of skin damage may have improved but it still may not have returned to normal. Through electron microscopy, it is found that in healed cases, the individual epidermis nuclei are comparatively large with collective chondriosome and obscure crista mitochondriales. It indicates that in cases that appear to be healed clinically, the microstructure of epidermal tissues hold features of pathological changes of cells before treatment. It shows that epidemic cells have not recovered, which may be a significant cause of its recurrence. If treatment is withdrawn right after the end of skin damage, it is susceptible to relapse. For this reason, treatment is recommended for another 2-3 months after being healed clinically to reduce the rate of relapse.

Insight from Empirical Wisdom

There are many methods to treat psoriasis, and a number of effective, simple and empirical formulas have been proven during years of clinical practice. They can be differentiated and categorized according to blood-heat, blood dryness, blood stasis, damp-heat and toxic heat.

The treatment principles are clearing heat to cool blood, enriching blood to moisten dryness, invigorating blood to remove stasis and removing dampness and resolving toxins. The clinical medications are summarized as follows:

(1) Application of Medicinals with the Actions of Invigorating Blood to Remove Stasis

Patients of psoriasis often have scaly skin or punctate hemorrhage after removing the scales. 35% of the patients have signs of a purple tongue body with macule stasis, buckling of skin capillary vessels when tested under a microscope, increased viscosity, and obviously increased vasopermeability. So clinically the method of invigorating blood to remove stasis is thought highly of, and satisfactory therapeutic effects have been achieved. For example, Zhou Ming-qi prescribed *Yín Xiè Bìng Huà Yū Tāng* (银屑病化瘀汤) to treat stubborn psoriasis and got great results. Ingredients: *é zhú* (Rhizoma Curcumae) 20g, *sān léng* (Rhizoma Sparganii) 10g, *jī xuè téng* (Caulis Spatholobi) 40g, *chì sháo* (Radix Paeoniae Rubra) 15g, *hóng huā* (Flos Carthami) 10g, *wēi líng xiān* (Radix et Rhizoma Clematidis) 15g, *wú gōng* (Scolopendra) 3 strips (take after grinding to a powder), *bái xiān pí* (Cortex Dictamni) 20g, *chán tuì* (Periostracum Cicadae) 10g, *huáng qí* (raw Radix Astragali) 40g, *shēng dì huáng* (Radix Rehmanniae Recens) 30g, *shēng gān cǎo* (raw Radix et Rhizoma Glycyrrhizae) 10g.

(2) Application of Medicinal Insects

Psoriasis is very obstinate and hard to cure completely because of toxic pathogens retained in the skin and interstitial spaces. In the clinic, doctors use medicinals from insects to treat the pathogens. This is a strategy similar to "fighting toxins with toxins". Insects medicinals enter the collaterals and are good at eliminating toxicity and wind. Extraordinary effects can often be achieved. Shi Xiang-rong created *Wū*

Shé Qīng Yǐn (乌蛇清饮), consisting of *wū shāo shé* (Zaocys) 20-30g, *quán xiē* (Scorpio) 5-10g, *fēng fáng* (Nidus Vespae) 10g, *chán tuì* (Periostracum Cicadae) 10g, *kǔ shēn* (Radix Sophorae Flavescentis) 15g, *bái xiān pí* (Cortex Dictamni) 15g, *jīn yín huā* (Flos Lonicerae)15g, *mǔ dān pí* (Cortex Moutan) 15g, *chì sháo* (Radix Paeoniae Rubra) 15g, *hé shǒu wū* (raw Radix Polygoni Multiflori) 15-30g, and *shēng gān cǎo* (raw Radix et Rhizoma Glycyrrhizae) 10g. He obtained good results.

(3) Application of Antitumor Drugs with the Action of Clearing Heat and Resolving Toxins

The origin of the disease is caused by viral and bacterial factors and has the feature of epidemic cells hypermultiplication. Therefore, one way of treating psoriasis is to prescribe medicinals which inhibit DNA construction and the generation of epidemic cells. This can be done in conjunction with controlling infections on the basis of syndrome differentiation. Chen Da-can created *Xiāo Bì Tāng* (消 疕 汤), consisting of *shuǐ niú jiǎo* (Cornu Bubali) 20-50g, *bái huā shé shé cǎo* (Herba Hedyotis) 30g, *shí shàng bǎi* (Herba Selaginellae Doederleinii) 15g, *hǔ zhàng* (Rhizoma et Radix Polygoni Cuspidati) 15g, *pú gōng yīng* (Herba Taraxaci) 15g, *bàn zhī lián* (Herba Scutellariae Barbatae) 6-9g, *dān shēn* (Radix et Rhizoma Salviae Miltiorrhizae) 15g, *xuán shēn* (Raidix Scrophulariae) 12g, and *tǔ fú líng* (Rhizoma Smilacis Glabrae) 30-50g. This formula can achieve good therapeutic effects.

Summary

Psoriasis is a chronic and recurrent dermatologic disease with many relapses and is hard to cure. The etiological factors are unclear. Treating from the perspective of blood has become a developing direction and a leading trend in the current treatment of psoriasis with Chinese medicine. Zhu Ren-kang thinks heat in the blood level is the major cause of psoriasis. Zhao Bing-nan advocates that psoriasis is blood heat. Qin

Wan-zhang and Wu Shao-xi look at the basis of psoriasis from another perspective in that it belongs to a blood stasis syndrome. They found, through substantial research of psoriasis, red blood cell deformation and abnormality of membrane ATP activity. This indicates obvious abnormalities of membrane function and even unusual membrane structure of the red blood cells. Gu Bo-hua considers that the main cause of psoriasis is blood deficiency, as it is always caused by a loss of nutritive blood generating wind and dryness which then fails to nourish the skin.

Psoriasis is characterized by its long disease course and recurrence so there is no method to cure psoriasis completely so far. Some biomedicinal drugs such as antitumor drugs and adrenal cortex hormones aim directly at a certain pathogenic links and can relieve symptoms but fail to achieve a complete cure. Side effects usually appear with the long-term use of medication. There are many Chinese medicinal treatments and the corresponding formulas and medicinals can be summarized as treating both interior and exterior.

In recent years, a number of effective Chinese patent capsules and pills have been explored such as *Kè Yín Wán* (克银丸) and *Yín Xiè Qīng Dài Wán* (银屑青黛丸). Initial empirical studies have also been done about them. For instance, *léi gōng téng* (Caulis Tripterigum Wilfordii) and its modified prescriptions are generally acknowledged to be effective in treating psoriasis. But many clinical reports examine simple formulas, empirical formulas or secret formulas. These are limited in individual cases or retrospective summaries with poor reproducibility. Therefore, systematic, scientific and prospective studies should be carried out further. However, the superiority of Chinese medicine treatment is not to be ignored in light of its clear therapeutics effect and fewer side effects.

In the future, we should open our minds. We should prescribe Chinese medicinals with the pharmacological actions of antitumor and inhibiting hyperplasy, based on treatments with pattern differentiation. This can improve the body constitution of patients, enhance healing rates and shorten the therapeutic course. Meanwhile, we should search for highly effective formulas and medicinals for treating psoriasis and find its causative mechanisms. We should further explore a number of new Chinese medicinal drugs of high effectiveness with little or no side effects.

SELECTED QUOTES FROM CLASSICAL TEXTS

Treatise on the Causes and Manifestations of Disease - Manifestations of Pyocutaneous Disease (诸病源候论·疮疡诸侯, *Zhū Bìng Yuán Hòu Lùn·Chuāng Yáng Zhū Hòu*):

干癣，但有匡郭，皮枯瘙痒，搔之白屑出是也。

"Dry psoriasis is characterized by obvious withering, dry skin and itching, white scales after scratching."

Standards of Diagnosis and Treatment - Surgeon (证治准绳·疡医, *Zhèng Zhì Zhǔn Shéng ·Yáng Yī*):

遍身起如风疹疥丹之状，其色白不痛，但搔痒抓起白疕，名曰蛇虱。

"Manifests by the appearance of urticaria and scabies all over the body, white in color without pain but with white scales after scratching. This is called *She Shi* (ichthyosis)."

Great Achievement of Surgery - Vol. Four - Ichthyosis (外科大成·卷四·白疕, *Wài Kē Dà Chéng · Juàn Sì·Bái Bì*):

白疕，肤如疹疥，色白而痒，搔起白疕，俗称蛇虱，由风邪客于皮肤，血燥不能荣养所致，宜搜风顺气丸，神应养真丹加白蛇之类。

"Psoriasis appears on the skin as urticaria and scabies with a white color and itching. There are white scales after being scratched. It is commonly called ichthyosis. It is caused by wind pathogens attacking the skin and blood dryness failing to nourish the skin. It is best to prescribe drugs as *Sōu Fēng Shùn Qì Wán* (搜风顺气丸) and *Shén Yīng Yǎng Zhēn Dān* (神应养真丹) and adding *bái huā shé* (Bungarus Parvus)."

Whole Book for Syndrome Differentiation and Treatment of Surgery ·Vol Four ·Syndrome of Indefinite Occurrence (外科证治全书 · 卷四 · 发无定处证 , *Wài Kē Zhèng Zhì Quán Shū·Juàn Sì·Fā Wú Dìng Chù Zhèng*):

白疕，一名疕风，皮肤干燥瘙痒，起如疹疥而色白。搔之屑起，渐至肢体枯燥干裂，血出痛楚，十指间皮厚而莫能搔痒。金太过，至秋深燥金用事，乃得此证。多患于血虚体瘦之人，生血润肤饮主之。用生猪脂搽之。

"Psoriasis is also called wind-ichthyosis and manifests as dry skin, itching, urticaria and scabies at the beginning of the disease and is white in color. Scales emerge after scratching, gradually developing to dry, parched, chapped skin on the limbs, pain after bleeding, thick skin between the fingers and severe itching. The disease is caused by "excessive metal in late autumn". It is usually seen in people with blood deficiency and frail, weak bodies. Formula: *Shēng Xuè Rùn Fū Yǐn* (生血润肤饮). Use pig oil ointment for external use."

The Golden Mirror of Medicine - Mental Cultivation Methods and Significance Trick of Surgery (医宗金鉴 · 外科心法要诀 , *Yī Zōng Jīn Jiàn·Wài Kē Xīn Fǎ Yào Jué*):

白疕，此证俗名蛇虱，生于皮肤，形如疹疥，色白而痒，搔起白皮。由风邪塞于皮肤，血燥不能营养所致。初服防风通圣散，次服搜风顺气丸，以猪脂、苦杏仁等分共捣，绢包擦之俱效。

"Psoriasis's folk name is *She Shi*. It occurs on the skin, shaped like measles and scabies rash, white in color and with itching. There are white scales after scratching. It is caused by wind pathogens blocking the skin, blood dryness failing to nourish the skin. Initially take *Fáng Fēng Tōng Shèng Sǎn* (防风通圣散), then take *Sōu Fēng Shùn Qì Wán* (搜风顺

气丸). Use equal amounts of pig fat and *kǔ xìng rén* (Semen Armeniacae Amarum) ground and wrapped with a cloth, then apply on the affected parts."

MODERN RESEARCH

Clinical Research

1. Pattern Differentiation and Corresponding Treatment

(1) Zhang Bing-zheng classified 35 cases of ordinary psoriasis into three types based on pattern differentiation: blood heat, blood dryness and blood stasis. Make observations of the blood after treatment. Basic formula: *bái huā shé shé cǎo* (Herba Hedyotis), *bàn zhī lián* (Herba Scutellariae Barbatae), *tǔ fú líng* (Rhizoma Smilacis Glabrae), *dān shēn* (Radix et Rhizoma Salviae Miltiorrhizae), *fēng fáng* (Nidus Vespae), *chuān xiōng* (Rhizoma Chuanxiong).

For a blood heat pattern, the treatment principles are clearing heat, cooling blood, resolving toxins and removing stasis, add *zǐ cǎo* (Radix Arnebiae), *shān dòu gēn* (Radix et Rhizoma Sophorae Tonkinensis) and *chì sháo* (Radix Paeoniae Rubra) to the basic formula.

For a blood dryness pattern, add *shēng dì huáng* (Radix Rehmanniae Recens), *huáng jīng* (Rhizoma Polygonati), *tiān mén dōng* (Radix Asparagi) and *jī xuè téng* (Caulis Spatholobi) to the basic formula to tonify yin, enrich blood and moisten skin.

For blood stasis, add *sān léng* (Rhizoma Sparganii), *é zhú* (Rhizoma Curcumae), *táo rén* (Semen Persicae), *hóng huā* (Flos Carthami) and *dān shēn* (Radix et Rhizoma Salviae Miltiorrhizae) to the basic formula to activate blood, promote qi circulation and transform stasis.

It is revealed that not every patient had a microcirculation disturbance. Patients with a blood stasis pattern had the most obvious change in microcirculation, patients of blood dryness pattern the second and patients of blood heat changed little. Blood tests according to Chinese medicine pattern differentiation of psoriasis indicated no regularity.

In addition, after treatment by Chinese medicine syndrome differentiation, after a decrease in damage or fundamental recovery of skin damage, the blood abnormalities recovered at equal pace. This indicates that doctors of Chinese medicine should insist on treatment by syndrome differentiation, and not rely on a fixed formula or medicinal. [1]

(2) Zhu Ren-kang divided psoriasis into two categories

For a blood heat and wind dryness pattern, treat by cooling blood, clearing heat and resolving toxins. Use *tǔ fú líng* (Rhizoma Smilacis Glabrae) 30g, *shān dòu gēn* (Radix et Rhizoma Sophorae Tonkinensis) 10g, *zǐ hé chē* (Placenta Hominis) 30g and *bái xiān pí* (Cortex Dictamni) 30g.

For a blood deficiency and wind dryness pattern, the treatment principles are tonifying yin, enriching blood and moistening dryness, assisted by resolving toxins. Use *shēng dì huáng* (Radix Rehmanniae Recens) 30g, *xuán shēn* (Raidix Scrophulariae) 30g, *dān shēn* (Radix et Rhizoma Salviae Miltiorrhizae) 30g, *huǒ má rén* (Semen Cannabis) 10g, *kǔ shēn* (Radix Sophorae Flavescentis) 10g and *shān dòu gēn* (Radix et Rhizoma Sophorae Tonkinensis). [2]

(3) Wang Ya-juan thought the etiology of psoriasis was blood heat, blood stasis, loss of nutritive blood and malnourishment of the skin, along with blood stasis. These play an important role in the generation and development of psoriasis.

In the initial stage of psoriasis, it is dominated by blood heat and excessive toxicity, for a chronic condition of dryness and consuming yin, so ordinary psoriasis is classified as patterns of blood heat, blood stasis and blood dryness for treatment. Created *Huó Xuè Tōng Luò Tāng* (活血通络汤) to treat 80 cases, the effective rate was 97.5%. [3]

(4) Han Yong-qun considered that psoriasis was caused by insufficient Kidney yin, deficient Spleen qi and external pathogenic toxic

heat invading the body.

Chronic toxic heat constraint can easily impair yin and blood. Insufficient yin and blood results in an unsmooth flow of blood, stagnant blood blocking the interior which fails to nourish the skin. This creates both deficiency and excess syndromes with yin deficiency, stasis and heat, and the appearance of dryness, heat, stasis and toxicity. The treatment principles are tonifying yin and clearing heat, resolving toxins and removing stasis. Used *Zǐ Yīng Tāng* (紫英汤) to treat 106 cases. The effective rate was 94.34%. [4]

2. Specific Formulas

(1) Dang Qian-li prescribed *Fù Fāng Qīng Dài Jiāo Náng* (复方青黛胶囊) to treat ordinary psoriasis, consisting of 14 Chinese medicinals such as *qīng dài* (Indigo Naturalis), *bái zhǐ* (Radix Angelicae Dahuricae), *tǔ fú líng* (Rhizoma Smilacis Glabrae), *zǐ cǎo* (Radix Arnebiae) and *dān shēn* (Radix et Rhizoma Salviae Miltiorrhizae). Functions to clear heat and resolve toxins, transform stasis to remove ecchymoses, and dispel wind to relieve itching. It demonstrated that the formula could improve various symptoms of ordinary psoriasis. Examination of the symptoms before and after treatment showed much improvement, all above 90%, without obvious side effects. [5]

(2) Zhang Xiang-de established *Liáng Xuè Yù Fēng Tāng* (凉血愈风汤) along with *Fù Fāng Dān Shēn Zhù Shè Yè* (复方丹参注射液) obtained good results in treating psoriasis.

Ingredients: *shēng dì huáng* (Radix Rehmanniae Recens) 30g, *shēng huái huā* (raw Flos Sophorae) 30g, *kǔ shēn* (Radix Sophorae Flavescentis) 30g, *tǔ fú líng* (Rhizoma Smilacis Glabrae) 50g, *bái xiān pí* (Cortex Dictamni) 30g, *cì jí lí* (Fructus Trbuli) 20g, *zào jiǎo cì* (Spina Gleditsiae) 12g, *wēi líng xiān* (Radix et Rhizoma Clematidis) 15g, *quán xiē* (Scorpio) 5g, *shé tuì* (Periostracum Serpentis) 5g, *gān cǎo* (Radix and Rhizoma

Glycyrrhizae) 9g, one dose a day, decoct in water for oral use.

For wind heat and blood heat, add *chì sháo* (Radix Paeoniae Rubra) 15g and *mŭ dān pí* (Cortex Moutan) 12g.

For constipation, add *shēng dà huáng* (raw Radix et Rhizoma Rhei) 12g and *zhĭ shí* (Fructus Aurantii Immaturus) 12g.

For sore throat and swelling, add *xuán shēn* (Raidix Scrophulariae) 15g and *shān dòu gēn* (Radix et Rhizoma Sophorae Tonkinensis) 12g.

For wind heat and damp-heat, add *huáng băi* (Cortex Phellodendri) 15g and *lóng dăn căo* (Radix Gentianae) 12g.

For wind heat and toxicity retention, add *huáng lián* (Rhizoma Coptidis) 6g and *zhī zĭ* (Fructus Gardeniae) 12g.

Used with *Fù Fāng Dān Shēn Zhù Shè Yè* (复方丹参注射液) 60-100ml diluted by 5% glucose solution for slow intravenous drip, once a day. After treatment, hemorheology and kallikrein microcirculation had improved. [6]

(3) Sun Li-yun prescribed *Liáng Xuè Huó Xuè Jiāo Náng* (凉血活血胶囊) to treat psoriasis in the active stage, which consisted of 13 Chinese medicinals such as *zĭ căo* (Radix Arnebiae), *qiàn căo* (Radix et Rhizoma Rubiae), *huái huā* (Flos Sophorae), *shān dòu gēn* (Radix et Rhizoma Sophorae Tonkinensis), *bái máo gēn* (Rhizoma Imperatae), *mŭ dān pí* (Cortex Moutan) and *dān shēn* (Radix et Rhizoma Salviae Miltiorrhizae).

Comparing the control group for random contract, double-blind contrast and clinical research. Conclusion: the healing rate of treatment group was 10%, the effective rate was 52.5% and the total effective rate was 62.5%. The healing rate of contrast group was 3.9%. The effective rate was 42.3%, and the total effective rate was 46.2%. The total effective rate of *Liáng Xuè Huó Xuè Jiāo Náng* (凉血活血胶囊)was much higher than contrast rate.

Liáng Xuè Huó Xuè Jiāo Náng (凉血活血胶囊) could obviously improve symptoms of itching, dry mouth and lips, dysphoria, irritation, constipation and scanty brownish urine of psoriasis with a blood heat pattern.[7]

(4) Wu Sheng-li prescribed *Jiě Dú Huà Yū Tāng* (解毒化淤汤): *shēng dì huáng* (Radix Rehmanniae Recens) 30g, *chì sháo* (Radix Paeoniae Rubra) 9g, *mǔ dān pí* (Cortex Moutan) 9g, *bǎn lán gēn* (Radix Isatidis) 30g, *shān dòu gēn* (Radix et Rhizoma Sophorae Tonkinensis) 9g, *bá qiā* (Rhizoma Smilacis Chinae) 30g, *shǔ yáng quán* (Herba Salani Septemlobi) 30g, *zé qī* (Herba Euphorbiae Helioscopiae), *tǔ fú líng* (Rhizoma Smilacis Glabrae) 30g, *kǔ shēn* (Radix Sophorae Flavescentis) 15g, *dān shēn* (Radix et Rhizoma Salviae Miltiorrhizae) 30g, to treat 50 cases of ordinary psoriasis and observed the therapeutic effect clinically and established psoriasis animal model with mouse tail, observing its influence on formation of granular cells of the mouse tail. The healing rate was 42.00%, and the total effective rate was 90.00%.

Jiě Dú Huà Yū Tāng (解毒化淤汤) is an effective prescription of treating ordinary psoriasis, which may relate to regulation of autoimmunity and inhibition of epidemic cells hyperplasia. Animal experiments showed *Jiě Dú Huà Yū Tāng* (解毒化淤汤) could conspicuously increase epidermatic granular layers of mouse tail scales, inferring that *Jiě Dú Huà Yū Tāng* (解毒化淤汤) took effect through inhibiting epidermatic cells hyperplasy, transforming parakeratotic cells to keratinocytes. [8]

(5) Peng Yong-nian gave emotional counseling with modified *Sì Wù Tāng* (四物汤) to treat severe ordinary psoriasis. At the initial visit, he inquired about the patient's history in detail, and found out whether or not significant events had happened in the patients' lives or work before or during the disease, and if there were psychological changes and stress suffered by them after attacks of psoriasis. He then conducted a psychological conversation with patients for no less than half an hour. The formula was based on *Sì Wù Tāng* (四物汤) [*dāng guī* (Radix Angelicae Sinensis), *shēng dì huáng* (Radix Rehmanniae Recens), *chì sháo*

(Radix Paeoniae Rubra), *chuān xiōng* (Rhizoma Chuanxiong)].

For the active stage, add medicinals such as *tǔ fú líng* (Rhizoma Smilacis Glabrae), *huái huā* (Flos Sophorae), *zǐ cǎo* (Radix Arnebiae), *mǔ dān pí* (Cortex Moutan) and *huáng qín* (Radix Scutellariae). For people of older age or patients in the stable stage, add herbs such as *huáng qí* (Radix Astragali), *dǎng shēn* (Radix Codonopsis) and *dān shēn* (Radix et Rhizoma Salviae Miltiorrhizae), one dose a day, decoct in water for oral use. The program had achieved satisfactory results, which avoided the application of drugs with strong side effects, and protected patient's health. [9]

(6) Feng Jing-chun treated serious psoriasis (erythrodermia pattern, agria pattern, arthropathia pattern) with *Léi Gōng Téng Duō Dài* (雷公藤多甙) and achieved good results. The author thought the Tripterygium Wilfordii prescription has positive effects in treating various pattern of serious psoriasis. It has the advantages of quick efficacy, fewer side effects and convenience, so *léi gōng téng* (Caulis Tripterigum Wilfordii) can be selected initially to treat cases with a short course of the disease and untreated by corticosteroid hormone and immune depressants. But periodic rechecks of urinary functions (hematuria) and hepatic and renal functions are needed. [10]

Jiang explored the mechanism of *léi gōng téng* (Caulis Tripterigum Wilfordii) in treating psoriasis, indicating that *léi gōng téng* (Caulis Tripterigum Wilfordii) inhibited the hyperplasy of ABKMA model epithelial cells, which may relate to its function of prohibiting secretion of cell factors. [11]

(7) Zheng Mao-rong prescribed *Kàng Yín Jiāo Náng Sān Hào* (抗银胶囊3号) which contained baicalin and powdered extract of rhababerone to treat psoriasis, achieving better results than prescribing baicalin alone with the total effective rate of 97.78%. Analyzing the mechanism, it is related to the action of baicalin to decrease the chematropism of PMN to leucotriene B4. In addition, it may connect with antibacterial and

immunosuppressive functions of rhababerone powdered extract. [12]

(8) Wang Bao-ting prescribed *Dí Yín Piàn* (迪银片) with *Fù Fāng Qīng Dài Wán* (复方青黛丸) to treat ordinary psoriasis in 30 cases, and healed 8 cases, healed basically 10 cases, 4 cases effective and improved 6 cases. The healing rate was 60.0%. The total effective rate was 73.3%. Both rates were higher than the *Dí Yín Piàn* (迪银片) comparison group. [13]

(9) Lu Ming-ren prescribed *Xiāo Xuǎn Miè Yín Tāng* (消癣灭银汤) to treat psoriasis in 500 cases, with the total effective rate of 97%. Ingredients: *chán tuì* (Periostracum Cicadae) 10g, *wú gōng* (Scolopendra) 2 stripes, *quán xiē* (Scorpio) 10g, *líng xiāo huā* (Flos Campsis) 30g, *shé tuì* (Periostracum Serpentis) 6g, *měi dēng mù* (Caulis Mayteni) 15g, *dān shēn* (Radix et Rhizoma Salviae Miltiorrhizae) 30g, *fáng fēng* (Radix Saposhnikoviae) 9g, *kǔ shēn* (Radix Sophorae Flavescentis) 15g. [14]

(10) Liu Guo-yan reported to have prescribed *Huái Xiāng Wū Shé Chōng Jì* (槐香乌蛇冲剂) to treat 122 cases of psoriasis, with the total effective rate of 90%. The formula consisted of *tǔ fú líng* (Rhizoma Smilacis Glabrae), *léi gōng téng* (Caulis Tripterigum Wilfordii), *shēng dì huáng* (Radix Rehmanniae Recens), *shēng huái huā* (raw Flos Sophorae), *zǐ cǎo* (Radix Arnebiae), *dān shēn* (Radix et Rhizoma Salviae Miltiorrhizae), *chì sháo* (Radix Paeoniae Rubra), *jī xuè téng* (Caulis Spatholobi), *fáng fēng* (Radix Saposhnikoviae), *bái xiān pí* (Cortex Dictamni), *bái jí lí* (Fructus Trbuli), and *wū shāo shé* (Zaocys).[15]

(11) Huang He-wei treated 48 cases of psoriasis patients with *Huáng Qí Guì Zhī Tāng* (黄芪桂枝汤). Ingredients: *huáng qí* (Radix Astragali) 30g, *dāng guī* (Radix Angelicae Sinensis) 15g, *guì zhī* (Ramulus Cinnamomi) 10g, *fáng fēng* (Radix Saposhnikoviae) 10g, *lián qiào* (Fructus Forsythiae) 12g, *gān cǎo* (Radix et Rhizoma Glycyrrhizae) 10g.

In clinical observation, they found that prescribing *huáng qí* (Radix Astragali) with *guì zhī* (Ramulus Cinnamomi) to treat psoriasis, satisfactory therapeutic effects could be expected, with the healing rate of 67% and effective rate of 83.7%. Compared to other therapies, it could shorten treatment courses, with quicker recovery of skin damage, no evident side effects and reduce the recurrence rate. [16]

(12) Wan Yan prescribed Chinese patent medicine *Huǒ Bǎ Huā Gēn Piàn* (火把花根片) which was developed by Sichuan Institute of Chinese Materia Medica to treat ordinary psoriasis, achieving good efficacy, with the healing rate of 56.95% and the total effective rate of 88.25%. [17]

(13) He Ling prescribed *Niú Huáng Chōng Jì* (牛黄冲剂) [Condensed granules consisting of medicinals as *shuǐ niú jiāo* (Cornu Bubali), *shēng dà huáng* (raw Radix et Rhizoma Rhei), *tǔ fú líng* (Rhizoma Smilacis Glabrae), *mǔ dān pí* (Cortex Moutan), *shēng dì huáng* (Radix Rehmanniae Recens), *bái huā shé shé cǎo* (Herba Hedyotis), *chì sháo* (Radix Paeoniae Rubra), *dāng guī* (Radix Angelicae Sinensis), *kǔ shēn* (Radix Sophorae Flavescentis), *bái xiān pí* (Cortex Dictamni), *shān dòu gēn* (Radix et Rhizoma Sophorae Tonkinensis), *shēng gān cǎo* (raw Radix and Rhizoma Glycyrrhizae), *jīn yín huā* (Flos Lonicerae) and *jú huā* (Flos Chrysanthemi)].

In treating 59 cases of ordinary psoriasis, healed 11 cases, 26 cases having effect, 14 cases effective, the total effective rate was 86.4%. 18]

(14) Liu Li-hong prescribed his own *Xiāo Yín Yóu* (消 银 油) [30g each of *zǐ cǎo* (Radix Arnebiae), *kǔ shēn* (Radix Sophorae Flavescentis), *bái xiān pí* (Cortex Dictamni) and *huáng bǎi* (Cortex Phellodendri), 20g each of *dì yú* (Radix Sanguisorbae), *hóng huā* (Flos Carthami), *bái zhǐ* (Radix Angelicae Dahuricae), *wū shāo shé* (Zaocys), *wú gōng* (Scolopendra) one stripe, the above medicinals sink in 1000ml teel oil for one day, decoct by slow fire to all medicinals until turned yellow, filtrate through four layers of gauze, the filtration put into a bottle and preserved for use], spread on 2-3 times , 30 days for a treatment course.

In treating 68 cases of ordinary psoriasis, healed 13 cases, 32 cases taking effect, 15 cases effective, 8 cases ineffective, the total effective rate was 88.24%. [19]

3. Acupuncture and Moxibustion

(1) Liao Ji-fa treated 41 cases of psoriasis with acupuncture treatment

【Manipulation】

For damage of upper limbs, head and face, select LI 11, SJ 6 (*zhī gōu*), GB 20, LI 4, matching SP 10, SP 6.

For face region, add LI 20, SI 18 (*quán liáo*).

For skin damage in the lower limbs, select SP 10, SP 6, ST 36, matching SJ 6 and LI 11.

For generalized skin damage, select DU 14, LI 11, LI 4, SP 10 and SP 6.

Curing 25 cases, 11 cases taking effect, 5 cases effective. [20]

(2) Gu Wen-shan treated 25 cases of psoriasis with acupuncture treatment

The main points were divided to two groups, the first group: DU 14, BL 13, BL 17 (*gé shù*), or BL 16 (*dū shù*), GB 20, at the same time matching with plum blossom needles on the affected parts of the waist and back. The second group: *sì shén cōng* (四神聪), LI 11, SP 10, or ST 40 (*fēng lóng*), ST 36; at the same time matching with plum blossom in head, limbs and affected parts.

The two groups of main points were prescribed alternately every day, retain the needle for 15-20 min, and tap the erythema skin with dermal needle until slightly bleeding, then cupping after withdrawal of the needle. 10-15 days as a treatment course. 5-7 days between the two courses.

Healed 6 cases, 5 cases taking effect, improved 10 cases, 2 cases ineffective. [21]

(3) Zhou Xian-xian treated psoriasis with ear bleeding treatment

【Manipulation】

Choose one ear, apply between the upper part and middle part of the posterior. After routine sterilization, make two cuts (to the extent of bleeding) 3-4 mm long in either direction with the edge, and not hurting the cartilage, bleeding 4-5 drops.

For serious patients, let it bleed for more amount, then spread on the cuts some iodine tincture to prevent infection, and cover with sterilized bandage for 3-5 days. Later, apply the above treatment on the other ear, alternate between the two ears. Healing 3 cases, 10 cases improved. [22]

(4) Zhang Lian-cheng treated psoriasis with bloodletting therapy in Hua Tuo point

Apply standard sterilization on Hua Tuo point, puncturing from above with a NO.26 acupuncture needle, without retention, to the extent of slight bleeding. If there is no bleeding, clean and press with cotton balls until there is some. Perform once a day or every other day for 15 times as a course. Stop other therapies during bloodletting therapy.

The healing rate of treating ordinary psoriasis in the active stage was 94.7%. The effective rate was 53%, the healing rate in stationary stage was 84% and the effective rate was 16%. [23]

(5) Ma Ming-ke treated psoriasis with external ointments in conjunction with plum blossom acupuncture therapy

The external formula was 10g each of *shēng chuān wū* (raw Radix Aconiti), *xióng huáng* (Realgar) and *liú huáng* (Sulphur), seven pieces of both castor bean and *bā dòu* (Fructus Crotonis), *shēng cǎo wū* (raw Radix Aconiti Kusnezoffii) and *shēng chuān wū* (raw Radix Aconiti) are fried by strong fire, ground with other medicinals to a fine powder and soaked in 100g of vinegar for one week. Apply conventional sterilization on affected parts, tap with plum blossom needles from the outside to inside in a spiral pattern until the center is slightly bleeding. Wipe the blood off and spread the medicinals on, 4 times a day, tapping once every other day.

In treating 10 cases, in the short term, followed up for 5 years, only one case recurred. [24]

(6) Zhang needled the DU meridian and obtained good effects

【Method】

Primarily select DU 11 (*shén dào*) and DU 10 (*líng tái*).

【Point modifications】

➢ SP 10, SP 6, LI 11 and LI 14; for local lesion with thick scales.

Use an encircling therapy. The stainless steel needles are 1.0 mm in diameter and 0.5cm long for the main points but should not have extremely sharp for the needle tips.

Apply conventional sterilization on the points before the procedure. The patient should sit up straight with the forearms crossed in front of the chest, bow the head and drop the shoulders to tense the skin on the back. The doctor fixes the needling point with left hand, with 30 degree needling angle downward of the needle tip, quickly needle DU 11, apply horizontal needling subcutaneously to DU 10 with needle tip. Insert to about 3.33cm. There should be sinking, sore, numb and expanding sensations felt locally or in the two arms. Retain the needle for 40 minutes without turning. 20 min.

For point modifications, select the No.30 needles 6.66cm long.

Point combination Ⅰ: Sit up straight, apply conventional sterilization on points, with even reinforcing-reducing method, after arrival of qi, retain the needle for 20 minutes.

Point combination Ⅱ: With a needling angle of 15 degrees oblique inserting the needle 2-3cm away from affected parts, with needle tip pointing to the center of affected areas. Select 4-8 points according to the area of infection focus by reducing method, retain for 30-40 minutes.

The total effective rate was 95% with the healing rate of 60%, improving rate of 20%, utility rate of 15%, invalid rate of 5%. [25]

(7) Tian Yang-chun prescribed ear bleeding therapy to treat 12 cases of ordinary psoriasis, healing 3 cases, improving 5 cases and 3 cases invalid

Select 1 to 3 distinct veins on the posterior part of the ear. Select one vein each time. Draw several drops of blood with a three-edged needle, beginning from the distal-heart end of the vein with swift pricking blood therapy, then select ear points upper ear root, shenmen, helix1, helix2, helix3, helix4, adrenal gland, endocrine, brain stem, occiput and lung. Once a week, 10 times as a course, take a break of 2 weeks between two courses. [26]

(8) Luan Tian-qing prescribed Chinese medicinals combined with needling and cupping to treat 30 cases of psoriasis, with the total effective rate of 96.7%

Xiāo Yín Tāng (消银汤): *shēng dì huáng* (Radix Rehmanniae Recens), *mài mén dōng* (Raidix Ophiopogonis), *jīn yín huā* (Flos Lonicerae), *huáng qín* (Radix Scutellariae), *dāng guī* (Radix Angelicae Sinensis), *hóng huā* (Flos Carthami), *chì sháo* (Radix Paeoniae Rubra), *chán tuì* (Periostracum Cicadae), *bái jiāng cán* (Bombyx Batryticatus), *wū shāo shé* (Zaocys) and *gān cǎo* (Radix et Rhizoma Glycyrrhizae). Decoct in water for oral use. 3 times a day, 10 days as a course.

Needle plus cupping treatment:

【Main points】

DU 14, DU 12 and DU 10.

【Point combinations】

BL 13, BL 23, BL 40.

【Point selection principles】

Include all the main points. Select the point combinations according to the body constitution and pathogenetic condition of patients.

【Method】

Sit up straight, after point selection, apply swift pricking blood therapy with three-edged needle and then do cupping, 4-6 cuppings at a time, retain for 20 minutes. Once a day, successive 10 days as a course.

Zhang Lian-cheng treated psoriasis with bloodletting therapy on the Hua Tuo points. Conventional sterilization on the Hua Tuo points, prick with a No. 26 acupuncture needle from above down to bleed a little without retaining the needle. If no bleeding, clean and pinch the point with cotton balls to make it bleed a little, once a day or every other day, 15 times as a treatment course. Stop other therapies during bloodletting therapy. For ordinary psoriasis in the active stage, the healing rate came to 94.7%, the effective rate of 53%; for stable stage, the healing rate was 84% and the effective rate was 16%. [27]

(9) Catgut implantation at acupoints

Zhou Min used catgut implantation at the acupoints to treat 12 cases of psoriasis with the total effective rate of 100%. Catgut implantation points: Main points: LI 11 (bilateral), SP 10 (bilateral), ST 36 (bilateral), sometimes matching DU 14, BL 13 and SP6. Select 4-6 points a time [28].

Liu Wei-bin used catgut implantation at acupoint with chorda chirurgicalis soaked by Chinese medicinals to treat psoriasis, indicating that its therapeutic effect was higher than the control group, cell immunity improved conspicuously, especially CD3 and the ratio of CD4/CD8 increased evidently. [29]

Experimental Studies

(1) Cheng Bin-zhu discussed the relation between TNF-α level of psoriasis patients and syndrome differentiation, indicating that there was no significant difference between the TNF-α level of psoriasis patients and normal control group. But TNF-α level in patients of blood deficiency and wind dryness syndrome was significantly lower than normal control group and the blood heat pattern group, which revealed that TNF-α had

reference value to syndrome differentiation. [30]

(2) Zhang Chao-ming made hemorheology research on psoriasis patients. He classified the disease into wind-damp and blood dryness patterns, blood deficiency and wind dryness patterns, stasis obstructing skin patterns. It demonstrated that under various shear rates, the whole blood viscosity and akaryocyte rigidity index increased most, and the number rose in accordance with the above pattern differentiation. In pattern of stasis obstructing the skin, the number reached the highest point, indicating that patients of this kind had obvious microcirculation disturbance.

The rising of akaryocyte rigidity index indicates erythrocyte deformability hypofunction. The author considers that medicinal therapies for invigorating blood to remove stasis, which have functions of increasing erythrocyte deformability, could be prescribed to improve therapeutic effect. [31].

(3) Liu Hua-chang reported test consequences of erythrocyte deformability and ATP membrane enzyme activity of 32 cases of different psoriasis pattern and 30 cases of a healthy control group. Erythrocyte deformability weakened, Na^{+}-K^{+}-ATP enzyme activity increased, while Ca^{2+}-Mg^{2+}-ATP enzyme activity decreased.

The abnormal order was: blood stasis type > blood dryness pattern > blood heat type. It reveals that psoriasis indicates a blood stasis syndrome, providing objective information for pattern differentiation, which plays an important role in exploring etiopathogenesis and directing the Chinese medicine treatment of psoriasis. [32]

(4) Fas system and bcl-2 family are autogenes of regulating apoptosis, and expression products APo-1 and APo-2.7 of Fas system have actions of inducing and promoting apoptosis; while bcl-2 can prevent and inhibit apoptosis triggered by various factors and a prolong cell survival.

Wang Ji-wen compared lymphocytic apoptosis in psoriasis patients of different pattern, showing that the APo-1 and APo-2.7 levels in patients are evidently higher than that of a healthy control group, and with the order of blood heat pattern> blood stasis pattern>blood deficiency pattern. While the expression of peripheral blood lymphocytes in psoriasis patients was much lower than that of the healthy contrast group, it decreased in the order of blood deficiency, blood stasis, blood heat. Patients of different pattern differed in apoptosis of peripheral blood lymphocyte, which was related to the overall health of the qi. [33]

(5) Transforming growth factor β (TGFβ) is a kind of endocrine factor functioning to transform cell growth, which actions to induce the transformation of normal cells, inhibit proliferation and promote apoptosis of cultured malpighian cells, as well as inhibit hyperplasy and transferring of cultured vascular endothelial cell. Experiments indicate that TGFβ in psoriasis patients had reduced down-regulation function to malpighian cell proliferation, causing loss of control of proliferation, which was possessed by all patterns.

Moreover, psoriasis patients' TGFβ activity abnormality happened in the process of disease, so syndrome differentiation of Chinese medicine is a true reflection of the nature of disease. [34]

(6) Jiang Xiang-de made *Yǐn Xiè Líng Tú Mó Jì* (银屑灵涂膜剂) for external use to treat psoriasis, and compared it with *Ēn Lín Ruǎn Gāo* (蒽林软膏) in its therapeutic effect. The major components are *dà huáng* (Radix et Rhizoma Rhei) and *tǔ dà huáng* (Radix Rumicis Nepalensis), to clear toxic heat, cool blood and transform stasis. Animal experiments showed that it inhibited caryocinesis of mouse vaginal epithelial cells, increased squamae surface granular layers of mouse tail, changed epidermatic cutinized format, turned from parakeratosis to complete cuticularization formation of granule layers, which could correct parakeratosis and cure psoriasis. The clinical therapeutic effect is identical to *Ēn Lín Ruǎn Gāo* (蒽林软膏), without obvious side effects. [35]

(7) Chen Ying-wen used MTT detection method of proliferative

response of cell strain B_{99} to determine blood serum level before and after orally taking Ginaton and in different pathogenetic stages, as well as IL-6 level in mononuclearcell cultural blood serum. It was revealed that IL-6 level in patients generated by microcirculation and mononuclearcell was higher than that in normal people and was related to the extent of the disease course.

After taking Ginaton orally as treatment for 2-4 weeks, the blood serum level and IL-6 level had significant differences comparing with that of pre-therapy, indicating that Ginaton inhibited secretion of IL-6 directly or indirectly. [36]

(8) Qin Xiao-wei observed actions of *yín xìng yè* (Folium Ginkgo) influencing chemotactic response of heterophil granulocyte in psoriasis patients. Platelet activating factor (PAF) is a kind of phospholipin mediators of inflammation with strong effects. Squamae of skin damage in psoriasis patients had PAF activity, and the content was higher than that of normal people. PAF receptor exists at the surface of neutrophils. The binding of PAF receptors promotes neutrophil gathering in epiderm, resulting in psoriasis. Ginkgolide, the active component of *yín xìng yè* (Folium Ginkgo) could resist PAF activity, thereby inhibiting the expression of PAF activity and chemotactic response of neutrophil to epiderm. [37]

(9) Lu You-lu studied 17 Chinese medicinals of different densities influencing hyperplasy of human epidermal cell cultured in vitro. In experiments that used *shēng dì huáng* (Radix Rehmanniae Recens), *dāng guī* (Radix Angelicae Sinensis), *chuān xiōng* (Rhizoma Chuanxiong) and *chì sháo* (Radix Paeoniae Rubra) there was evident action of inhibiting epidermal cell proliferation, which confirmed that from a cellular level, as the basic components of modified *Sì Wù Tāng* (四物汤), they had clear effect in treating psoriasis. *Bái huā shé shé cǎo* (Herba Hedyotis), *mǔ dān pí* (Cortex Moutan), *é zhú* (Rhizoma Curcumae) and *hóng huā* (Flos

Carthami), as the additional components, had excellent inhibiting action, helping to improve the therapeutic effect. The experiment provided an experimental basis for approaches on the mechanisms of Chinese medicinals treating psoriasis. [38]

(10) Qin Wan-zhang applied methods of invigorating blood to transform stasis to treat psoriasis, with the internal use of *kūn míng shān hǎi táng* (Radix Tripterygii Hypoglaucii), *léi gōng téng* (Caulis Tripterigum Wilfordii) and activating blood prescription, determined cyclic nucleotide before and after treatment. Before treatment, cAMP decreased conspicuously, ratio of cAMP/cGMP also decreased; after treatment, the index increased or returned to normal with the improvement of damage, indicating that medicinals for invigorating blood to transform stasis function to regulate cyclic nucleotide metabolism. [39]

(11) Lin Xi-ran prescribed *Xǐ Shù Dīng* (喜 树 酊) to treat psoriasis, achieving good effect. He studied female sex hormone periodic vaginal epithelium mouse model, epidermal cell caryocinesis of mouse tail squamae and action of promoting forming of granular layer of epidermis. All of which indicate that the mechanism of *Xǐ Shù Dīng* (喜树酊) for treating psoriasis may have actions of inhibiting epidermal cell proliferation, and influencing process of cuticular cuticularization. [40] Ethanol tincture is ethanol, highly volatile, incentive and not adhering on skin, which influences its therapeutic effect. Wang Ai-min improved the dosage form to *Xǐ Shù Guǒ Tú Mó Jì* (喜 树 果 涂 膜 剂) (0.7611g camptothecin in one gram of plastics) to treat psoriasis, achieving a good effect. [41]

(12) Tian Di studied influence of four kinds of sophocarpidine (aloperine, sophocarpidine, ammothamnine and sophocarpine) on Colo16 cell proliferation, and explored mechanism of *kǔ shēn* (Radix Sophorae Flavescentis) treating psoriasis.

The experiments showed that aloperine at the density of 400mg/ml,

200mg/ml, 100mg/ml, and 50mg/ml could inhibit Colo16 cell proliferation, sophocarpidine and ammothamnine have inhibitory action at the density of 400mg/ml, and sophocarpine has no inhibitory action at any density, confirming that *kǔ shēn* (Radix Sophorae Flavescentis) actually has active constituent inhibiting epithelial cells growth. [42]

(13) Zhang Jun-ling determined the contents of subdiploid cell by flow cytometer, and applied method of DNA gragmentation analysis and annexin apoptosis detection, finding that ammothamnine has actions of increasing the contents of subdiploid cells, DNA gragmentation rate and phosphatidyl serine extramembranous of Malpighian cell. [43]

(14) Wu Jing-hai studied actions of tanshinol influencing cell adhesion molecule expression of peripheral blood mononuclear cell in psoriasis patients.

Immunohistochemistry researches had shown that, expression of many adhesion molecules such as FLA-1, ICAM-1 and VCAM-1 strengthened in Malpighian cells in skin damage area and surrounding areas of psoriasis patients in active stage. And the expressions in small vessels of dermal papilla and beneath papilla were higher than normal, which had positive correlation with the number of inflammatory infiltration inside the skin. Many soluble adhesion molecule level in blood serum of psoriasis patients rose also.

After peripheral blood mononuclear cell in psoriasis patients incubated with tanshinol, its adhesiveness with endothelial cell of human allantoic veins weakened, indicating that tanshinol has actions of inhibiting expression of adhesion molecule ICAM-1, which may take effect through actions of inhibiting adhesiveness of peripheral blood mononuclear cell with vascular endothelial cell. [44]

(15) Xiao Qing-lin researched the changes in blood panels after treating with different dosages of *dān shēn* (Radix et Rhizoma Salviae Miltiorrhizae). There were pathological abnormalities in red cell

aggregation intensifying and deformation decreasing. *Dān shēn* (Radix et Rhizoma Salviae Miltiorrhizae) had the function of dilating blood vessels, anticoagulation, invigorating blood to transform stasis and improving the above pathological phenomenon. The therapeutic effect of large dosage (60-100 ml) was superior to medium dosage (30-50 ml), and the medium dosage superior to small dosage (10-20 ml). [45]

(16) Liu Bo studied the anti-inflammatory and antiimmune actions of *Yín Xiè Líng* (银屑灵), which consisted of herbs such as *kǔ shēn* (Radix Sophorae Flavescentis), *bái xiān pí* (Cortex Dictamni) and *tǔ fú líng* (Rhizoma Smilacis Glabrae). These function to dispel wind and dry dampness, clear heat to resolve toxins and invigorate blood to transform stasis.

Pharmacological experiments showed that *Yín Xiè Líng* (银屑灵) had conspicuous actions of inhibiting mouse aural inflammation caused by croton oil, cavia cobaya syncope due to beta-imidazolyle thylamine, and mouse tardive allergies. In addition, it also resisted mouse itching caused by dextran, having anti-inflammatory and anti-immune actions. [46]

(17) Cheng Xue-hua studied the medication mechanism of *Yù Yín Piàn* (愈银片), consisting of *huái huā* (Flos Sophorae), *sōng zhǐ* (Pine Rosin), *dāng guī* (Radix Angelicae Sinensis), *mǔ dān pí* (Cortex Moutan), *shēng dì huáng* (Radix Rehmanniae Recens), *chuān xiōng* (Rhizoma Chuanxiong), *sān léng* (Rhizoma Sparganii) and *é zhú* (Rhizoma Curcumae). Studies showed that *Yù Yín Piàn* (愈银片) improved considerably the granular layer of epidermis formation in mouse tail, transforming aceratosis to complete cuticularization; inhibited basal cell caryocinesis of mouse vaginal mucosa, slowing down epidermal proliferation; and decreased itch-threshold to histamine phosphate, functioning to relieve itching, improving symptoms and finally curing psoriasis. [47]

(18) Gao Bing-ai prescribed *Fù Fāng Shēn Dì Tāng* (复方参地汤) with small dosages of *Dí Yín Piàn* (迪银片) to treat chronic psoriasis of

plaque pattern, and detected blood serum IL-8 level and blood plasma endothelin level before and after treatment of 11 cases. The index after treatment decreased conspicuously compared with pre-therapy. [48]

(19) Lou Wei-hai made clinical and experimental studies on psoriasis during active stage with *Liáng Xuè Huó Xuè Tāng* (凉血活血汤). *Liáng Xuè Huó Xuè Tāng* (凉血活血汤) was an empirical formula established by the late famous physician Zhang Zhi-li, consisting of medicinals such as *bái máo gēn* (Rhizoma Imperatae), *shēng dì huáng* (Radix Rehmanniae Recens), *zǐ cǎo* (Radix Arnebiae), *qiàn cǎo* (Radix et Rhizoma Rubiae), *bǎn lán gēn* (Radix Isatidis), *shān dòu gēn* (Radix et Rhizoma Sophorae Tonkinensis), *shú dà huáng* (Prepared Radix et Rhizoma Rhei) and *líng yáng jiǎo fěn* (Cornu Saigae Tataricae Pulveratum), treat psoriasis in active stage, achieving a very good effect.

The experiments showed that *Liáng Xuè Huó Xuè Tāng* (凉血活血汤) had actions of lowering levels of blood plasma thromboxan B_2, 6-ketone-prostaglandin F1α and blood resum interleukin-8 (IL-8), correcting arachidonic acid metabolism abnormality, inhibiting mediators of inflammation releasing and regulating body immune function. [49]

Li Wei-fan created experiments that showed *Liáng Xuè Huó Xuè Tāng* (凉血活血汤) could lower tumor necrosis factor-α (TNF-α) level in blood serum. After treating, levels of blood serum TNF-α and IL-8 lowered with improvement of pathogenetic conditions. [50]

(20) *Zhú Huáng Kē Lì* (竹黄颗粒) was an empirical formula from Professor Ou-yang Heng of Second Affiliated Hospital of Hunan Traditional Chinese Medicine College, consisting of medicinals such as *dàn zhú yè* (Folium Bamboo), *huáng qín* (Radix Scutellariae), *dǎng shēn* (Radix Codonopsis), *zhī zǐ* (Fructus Gardeniae), *shēng shí gāo* (Gypsum Fivrosum), *mài mén dōng* (Raidix Ophiopogonis), *huáng bǎi* (Cortex Phellodendri), *huáng lián* (Rhizoma Coptidis), *lòu lú* (Radix Rhapontici), and *shuǐ niú jiǎo* (Cornu Bubali), functioning to clear heat and resolve

toxins, benefit qi and enrich yin.

Blood serum interleukin-6 (IL-6) could induce and promote Malpighian cell hyperplasy, intensify T cells gathering intraepidermally, and promote inflammatory formation of psoriatic skin damage; tumor necrosis factor α (TNF-α) was an important inflammatory promoting cell factor, which had action of promoting inflammatory formation of psoriatic skin damage.

Yang Zhi-bo researched IL-6 and TNF-α levels before and after orally taking *Zhú Huáng Kē Lì* (竹黄颗粒) by psoriatic patients. It indicated that with the recovery of skin damage and clinical symptoms of the patients, IL-6 and TNF-α levels returned to normal. [51]

Luo Wen-hui studied the therapeutic efficacy of *Zhú Huáng Kē Lì* (竹黄颗粒) treating ordinary psoriasis and its influences on the blood. *Zhú Huáng Kē Lì* (竹黄颗粒) turned out to have good effect in treating ordinary psoriasis, which was worthy of being further explored. [52]

(21) Wang Ya-juan evaluated the clinical curative effects of *Zǐ Cǎo Huó Xuè Tāng* (紫草活血汤) in treating ordinary psoriasis and its influence on the blood. It was indicated that *Zǐ Cǎo Huó Xuè Tāng* (紫草活血汤) could lower patient's blood viscosity and was effective in the clinic. [53]

(22) Song Zhi-qi established mouse tail squamae epiderm—vaginal epithelium model, to research the influence on epidermal cuticularization, cell caryocinesis and proliferation, and proliferating cell nuclear antigen (PCNA) with *É Zhú Yóu Shuāng Jì* (莪术油霜剂) of different density applied externally.

It is indicated that *É Zhú Yóu Shuāng Jì* (莪术油霜剂) is a medicinal of external use of medium therapeutic effect, with probable mechanism of inhibiting Malpighian cell proliferation and promoting Malpighian cell differentiation. [54]

(23) Ma Xue-wei prescribed *Kè Yín Yī Hào Jiāo Náng* (克银 I 号胶囊) (Main ingredients: *zǐ cǎo* (Radix Arnebiae), *shuǐ niú jiǎo fěn* (Cornu

Bubali Pulveratum), *dà xuè téng* (Caulis Sargentodoxae), *hóng téng* (Caulis Sargentodoxae), *wú gōng* (Scolopendra), *quán xiē* (Scorpio), *chì sháo* (Radix Paeoniae Rubra), *mǔ dān pí* (Cortex Moutan), *dāng guī* (Radix Angelicae Sinensis)), to treat ordinary psoriasis in 40 cases, healing 29 cases, 9 cases effective, the therapeutic was higher than the *Fù Fāng Qīng Dài Wán* (复方青黛丸) group.

After treatment, epidermal growth factor (EGF) level lowered patients epiderm, indicating that *Kè Yín Yī Hào Jiāo Náng* (克银 I 号胶囊) had actions of weakening epidermal cell proliferative differentiation, relieving epidermal hyperkeratinization of skin damage, parakeratosi and dermic inflammatory cell infiltration, so as to enter recovery phase. [55]

(24) Lin Rui-fen made clinical and immunological studies on the folk recipe, *Sān Téng Tāng* (三 藤 汤) (*léi gōng téng* (Caulis Tripterigum Wilfordii), *shǒu wū téng* (Caulis Polygoni Multiflori), *jī xuè téng* (Caulis Spatholobi), *gān cǎo* (Radix and Rhizoma Glycyrrhizae)). The effective rate reached 90%, 65% having effect. After treatment CD_3、CD_4、CD_8 ascended, and ratio of CD_4/ CD_8 decreased, indicating that *Sān Téng Tāng* (三 藤 汤) could effectively improve immune dysfunctions. The author proposed to first choose *Sān Téng Tāng* (三藤汤) to treat patients who had not received corticosteroid hormone and immune depressant treatment. [56]

(25) Feng Jie applied immunohistochemistry method to detect epithelial cells c-myc expression in 30 cases of ordinary psoriasis treated by *Qīng Dài Jiāo Náng* (青 黛 胶 囊). Comparing 12 cases from a normal group, through statistical treatment, there was significant difference between the two groups in expression of skin damage, the expression of patients was much higher.

After curing, c-myc expression decreased, no significant difference was found comparing with contrast group. C-mcy expression in epithelial cells is evidently related to pathological changes of psoriasis, indicating that it takes effect by lowering cmyc expression in epithelial cells. The research provided experimental basis for *Fù Fāng Qīng Dài Jiāo Náng* (复方青黛胶囊) treating psoriasis. [57]

(26) Min Zhong-sheng studied the clinical therapeutic effect of Chinese medicinal steaming therapy in treating ordinary psoriasis, and made initial pharmacodynamic research of *Ài Bǎi Xūn Jì* (艾柏熏剂).

Treating 71 cases of ordinary psoriasis, observed the color of erythema, infiltration extent and changes of squamae and itching by integration; made pharmacodynamic experiments on *Ài Bǎi Xūn Jì* (艾 柏 熏 剂) with mouse vaginal epithelial cell caryocinesis detection and granule lay formation detection of mouse tail squamae. The effective rate was 56.34%. It functioned to eliminate erythema infiltration and squamae, and relieve itching. *Ài Bǎi Xūn Jì* (艾柏熏剂) could conspicuously inhibit caryocinesis of mouse vaginal epithelium and had therapeutic effect in parakeratosis. [58]

(27) Jiang Xiang-de prescribed *Yín Xiè Líng Tú Mó Jì* (银屑灵涂膜剂) externally and studied its influence on Vaginal epithelial cell caryocinesis of female sex hormone periodic Mus musculus albus and granular layer of epidermis formation of mouse tail squamae, finding that the therapeutic effect of *Yín Xiè Líng Tú Mó Jì* (银屑灵涂膜剂) was in accordance with *Ēn Lín Ruǎn Gāo* (蒽林软膏), but was superior in dosage form. [59]

(28) Yang Zhi-bo studied the influence of *Zhú Huáng Kē Lì* (竹 黄 颗 粒) on neuroendocrine function of psoriatic patients in active stage. It is indicated that *Zhú Huáng Kē Lì* (竹黄颗粒) had the action of regulating of neuroendocrine functional abnormality, thereby, improving patients quality of life. [60]

(29) Liu Ming researched the mechanism of *Xiāo Yín Jiě Dú Yǐn* (消银解毒饮) in treating psoriasis, finding that *Xiāo Yín Jiě Dú Yǐn* (消银解毒饮) in both large and small dosages could effectively resist SEB inducing IL-8. Combined with super antigen theory, from cell biology level, the action of *Xiāo Yín Jiě Dú Yǐn* (消银解毒饮) is well elaborated. [61]

REFERENCES

[1] Zhang Bing-zhen. Discussion on Relation between Pattern Differentiation and Hemorheology (银屑病中医分型与血液流变学关系探讨). *Chinese Journal of Dermatovenereology of Integrated Traditional And Western Medicine* (中西医结合皮肤性病学杂志). 1996, (11): 13.

[2] Zhu Ren-kang. Clinical Progress on *Kè Yín Fāng* in Treating Psoriasis (克银方治疗银屑病的临床研究进展). *Journal of Traditional Chinese Medicine* (中医杂志). 1983, 24(9): 31

[3] Wang Ya-juan, Dong Xi-lin, Chen Qi, et al. *Huó Xuè Tōng Luò Tāng* Treating Ordinary Psoriasis 80 Cases (活血通络汤治疗寻常型银屑病80例). *Shaanxi Journal of Traditional Chinese Medicine* (陕西中医). 2002, 23(9)：796.

[4] Han Yong-qun, Yuan Guang-qi, Zhu Lian-qing, et al. Discussion on Dependability of Treating Psoriasis from Yin Deficiency and Stagnated Heat and Hemorheology (从阴虚瘀热论治银屑病与血液流变学的相关性). *Shanxi Clinical Medicine Journal* (山西临床医药杂志). 2001, 10(4): 264.

[5] Dang Qian-li, Luo Xiu-rong, Ma Xiao-ping, et al. Therapeutic Effect Observation on *Fù Fāng Qīng Dài Jiāo Náng* Treating Ordinary Psoriasis (复方青黛胶囊治疗寻常型银屑病疗效观察). *Journal of Clinical Dermatology* (临床皮肤科杂志). 1999, 28(2): 115.

[6] Zhang Xian-de. Clinical Research of *Liáng Xuè Yù Fēng Tāng* with *Fù Fāng Dān Shēn Zhù Shè Yè* Treating Psoriasis (凉血愈风汤复方丹参注射液治疗银屑病的临床研究). *Chinese Journal of Dermatovenereology of Integrated Traditional and Western Medicine* (中西医结合皮肤性病学杂志). 1996, 11: 19.

[7] Sun Li-yun, Chen Kai, Deng Bing-rong, et al. Clinical Research of *Liáng Xuè Huó Xuè Jiāo Náng* Treating Psoriasis (凉血活血胶囊治疗血热型银屑病的I临床研究). *Chinese Journal of Dermatovenereology of Integrated Traditional and Western Medicine* (中国中西医结合皮肤性病学杂志). 2002, 1(1): 16.

[8] Wu Sheng-li, Xu Neng, Cheng Jian-ming, et al. Clinical and Experimental Study on *Jiě Dú Huà Yū Tāng* Treating Psoriasis (解毒化淤汤治疗银屑病的临床和实验研究). *Chinese Journal of Dermatology* (中华皮肤科杂志). 2004, 37(3): 133-134.

[9] Peng Yong-nian. Summary of Psychological Conversation *Matching Modified Sì Wù Tāng* in Treating Severe Ordinary Psoriasis 36 Cases (心理疏导并用中药四物汤加味治疗重症寻常型银屑病36例小结). *Chinese Journal of Dermatovenereology of Integrated Traditional And Western Medicine* (中西医结合皮肤性病学杂志). 1998, (12): 35.

[10] Feng Jing-chun. Clinical Analysis of Tripterygium Glycosides Treating Serious Psoriasis 13 Cases (雷公藤多甙治疗严重型银屑病13例临床分析). *Journal of Clinical*

Dermatology (临床皮肤科杂志). 1996, 25(4): 216.

[11] Jiang Yi-hua, Zheng Yi. Research on Tripterigum Wilfordii Decoction Influencing Psoriatic ABKMA Model (雷公藤煎液对银屑病 ABKMA 模型影响的研究). *Hubei Journal of Traditional Chinese Medicine* (湖北中医杂志). 2001, 23(6): 47-48.

[12] Zheng Mao-rong. Baicalin Influencing on Neutrophil and Chemotactic Response of Leukotriene B4 of Psoriasis Patients (黄芩甙对银屑病患者中性粒细胞对白三烯 B4 趋化反应的影响). *Journal of Clinical Dermatology* (临床皮肤科杂志). 1996, 25(3): 149.

[13] Wang Bao-ting, Li Ting-yi. Observation of Therapeutic Effect of *Dí Yín Piàn* Associating with *Fù Fāng Qīng Dài Wán* Treating Ordinary Psoriasis (迪银片联合复方青黛丸治疗寻常型银屑病疗效观察). *Chinese Journal of Dermotovenereolory* (中国皮肤性病学杂志). 2002, 16(3): 216.

[14] Lu Ming-ren, Lu Jun-fang, Lu Jun-ya. *Xiāo Xuǎn Miè Yín Tāng* Treating Psoriasis 500 Cases (消癣灭银汤治疗银屑病 500 例). *China's Naturopathy* (中国民间疗法). 2002, 10(2): 4.

[15] Liu Guo-yan, Xu Wen-hao. Therapeutic Effect Observation of *Huái Xiāng Wū Shé Chōng Jì* Treating Psoriasis 122 Cases (槐香乌蛇冲剂治疗银屑病 122 例临床疗效观察). *China Journal of Leprosy and Skin Disease* (中国麻风皮肤病杂志). 2002, 18(1): 59.

[16] Huang He-wei, Wu Hong-lin, Wu Pei-lin. Clinical Observation of *Huáng Qí Guì Zhī Tāng* Treating Psoriasis 48 Cases (黄芪桂枝汤治疗银屑病 48 例临床观察). *Journal of Changzhi Medical College* (长治医学院学报). 2003, (2): 145-146.

[17] Wang Yan, Wang Li-hua. Therapeutic Effect Observation of *Huǒ Bǎ Huā Gēn Piàn* Treating Ordinary Psoriasis (火把花根片治疗寻常型银屑病疗效观察). *Journal of Chinese Physician* (中国医师杂志). 2003, (S1): 2471.

[18] He Ling, Wu Song. Clinical Observation of *Niú Huáng Chōng Jì* Treating Ordinary Psoriasis 59 Cases (牛黄冲剂治疗寻常型银屑病 59 例临床观察). *Journal of Traditional Chinese Medicine* (中医杂志). 2002, 43(2): 123-124.

[19] Liu Li-hong. Self-made *Xiāo Yín Yóu* Treating Psoriasis 68 Cases (自制消银油治疗银屑病 68 例). *Journal of External Therapy of Traditional Chinese Medicine* (中医外治杂志). 2003, 12(1): 48.

[20] Liao Ji-fa. Acupuncture Treatment of Psoriasis 41 Cases (针刺治疗银屑病 41 例). *Journal of Zhejiang College of Traditional Chinese Medicine* (浙江中医学院学报). 1981, (6): 47.

[21] Gu Xia-xian. Analysis of Acupuncture Treatment of Psoriasis 25 Cases (针刺治疗银屑病 25 例疗效分析). *Shanghai Journal of Acupuncture and Moxibustion* (上海针灸杂志). 1982, (3): 4.

[22] Zhou Xian-xian. Ear Acupoint Cutting Therapy of Psoriasis (耳穴割治治疗银屑

病). *Chinese Acupuncture and Moxibustion* (中国针灸). 1985. 5(2): 13.

[23] Zhang Lian-cheng. Hua Tuo Point Bloodletting Therapy of Psoriasis (华佗穴放血治疗银屑病). *Zhejiang Journal of Traditional Chinese Medicine* (浙江中医杂志). 1990, 25(9): 423.

[24] Ma Ming-ke. Drug for External Use Matching Pyonex Treating Psoriasis (外擦药配合梅花针治疗牛皮癣). *Sichuan Journal of Traditional Chinese Medicine* (四川中医). 1984, 2(1): 61.

[25] Zhang Jing-min. Clinical Observation of Round-sharp Needle Treating Psoriasis [J] (圆利针为主治疗银屑病临床观察 [J]). *Tianjin Journal of Traditional Chinese Medicine* (天津中医药). 2003, 20(4): 68.

[26] Tian Yang-chun. Ear Acupoint Cutting Therapy Treating Ordinary Psoriasis 12 Cases [J] (耳穴割治法治疗寻常型银屑病 12 例 [J]). *Chinese Acupuncture and Moxibustion* (中国针灸). 1998, 2: 113.

[27] Luan Tian-qing. Therapeutic Effect Observation of Chinese Medicinal Matching Needling and Cupping Treating 30 Cases of Psoriasis (中药合针罐治疗银屑病 30 例疗效观察). *China Journal of Traditional Chinese Medicine* (中医药学报). 2001, 29(5): 32.

[28] Liu Wei-bin, Zhang Kai. Acupoint Embeded with Chorda Chirurgicalis Soaked in Chinese Medicinal Treating Psoriasis and Its Influence on Immunity (中药浸泡羊肠线作穴位埋置治疗银屑病及其对免疫功能的影响). *Journal of Dermatology and Venerology* (皮肤病与性病). 2001, 23(3): 20-21.

[29] Zhou Min. Clinical Observation of Catgut Implantation at Acupoint Treating 200 Cases (穴位埋线治疗银屑病 200 例临床观察 [J]). *Journal of External Therapy of Traditional Chinese Medicine* (中医外治杂志). 1995, 2: 17.

[30] Cheng Bin-zhu. Initial Research of Relation between Blood Serum Tumor Necrosis Level and Syndrome of Psoriasis Patients (银屑病患者血清肿瘤坏死因子水平与中医辨证关系的初步研究). *Chinese Journal of Basic Medicine in Traditional Chinese Medicine* (中国中医基础医学杂志). 1999, 5(9): 42.

[31] Zhang Chao-ming, Zhang Yan-fei. Research on Hemorheology of Psoriatic Patients (银屑病患者的血液流变学研究). *Sichuan Journal of Traditional Chinese Medicine* (四川中医). 1999, 17(8): 9.

[32] Liu Hua-chang, Li Guan-yong, Qu Shen, et al. Relation between Pattern Differentiation of Psoriasis and Erythrocyte Deformability and Membrane ATP Enzyme Activity (银屑病辨证分型与红细胞变形能力及膜 ATP 酶活性的关系). *Chinese Journal of Integrated Traditional and Western Medicine* (中国中西医结合杂志). 1994, 14(4): 210.

[33] Wang Ji-wen, Liu Rui-xia, Liu Hua-chang, et al. Lympholeukocyte Apoptotic

Comparison among Different Patterns of Psoriatic Patients (银屑病患者不同证型间淋巴细胞凋亡的比较). *Journal of Shan dong University of Traditional Chinese Medicine* (山东中医药大学学报). 2000, 24(2): 114.

[34] Peng Zhen-hui, Zhang Mei-fang, Zhang Bing-zheng, et al. Bioassay of Blood Serum TGFβ TNF-α by Pattern Differentiation (银屑病中医分型血清 TGFβTNF-α 的生物测定). *The Chinese Journal of Dermatovenereology* (中国皮肤性病学杂志). 2000, 14(1): 2.

[35] Jiang Xiang-de, Li Jin, Wang Su-wen, et al. Experimental Study *of Yín Xiè Líng Tú Mó Jì* Treating Psoriasis (银屑灵涂膜剂治疗银屑病的实验研究). *Tianjin Journal of Traditional Chinese Medicine* (天津中医). 2002, 19(5): 39.

[36] Chen Ying-wen. IL-6 level Variation of Orally Taking Ginaton of Psoriatic Patients (银屑病患者口服银杏叶提取物治疗中 IL-6 水平变化). *Chinese Journal of Dermatovenereology of Integrated Traditional And Western Medicine* (中西医结合皮肤性病学杂志). 1996, (11): 31.

[37] Qin Xiao-wei, Zheng Mao-rong, Mou Xian-long, et al. Influence of Folium Ginkgo on Neutrophil Chemotactic Response of Psoriatic Patients (银杏叶对银屑病患者中性粒细胞趋化反应的影响). *Journal of Clinical Dermatology* (临床皮肤科杂志). 1998, 27(6): 154.

[38] Lu You-lu. Seventeen Chinese Medicinals Influencing on Cultural Epidermal Cell Proliferation (17 味中药对培养的表皮细胞增殖的影响). *Journal of Clinical Dermatology* (临床皮肤科杂志). 1996, 25(4): 202.

[39] Qin Wang-zhang. Clinical Observation and Mechanism Approach of *Sān Téng Táng Jiāng* Treating 371 Cases of Dermatologic Disease (三藤糖浆治疗 371 例皮肤病临床观察及其机理探讨). *Collected Research Papers of the 2nd Conference of Dermatovenereology Committee of Chinese Association of the Integration of Traditional and Western Medicine* (中国中西医结合学会皮肤性病专业委员会第二届学术会议论文汇编). 1987, (7): 99.

[40] Lin Xi-ran. Research on *Xǐ Shù Dīng* Treating Psoriasis (喜树酊治疗银屑病的研究). *National Medical Journal of China* (中华医学杂志). 1987, 67(1): 4.

[41] Wang Ai-min, Liu Zhen-fu, Liu Sheng-you, et al. *Xǐ Shù Guǒ Tú Mó Jì* Treating Psoriasis (喜树果涂膜剂治疗银屑病). *Journal of Clinical Dermatology* (临床皮肤科杂志). 1998, 27(4): 243.

[42] Tian Di, Qin Jian-zhong. Four Kinds of Radix Sophorae Flavescentis Alkloid Influencing on Human Epithelial Cells Proliferation (四种苦参生物碱对人角朊细胞增殖的影响). *Chinese Journal of the Practical Chinese with Modern Medicine* (实用中西医结合杂志). 1997, 10(11): 1110.

[43] Zhang Jun-ling, Chen Xue-rong, Yin Jin-zhu. Research on Ammothamnine Inducing Malpighian Cell Apoptosis (氧化苦参碱诱导角质形成细胞凋亡研究). *The*

Chinese Journal of Dermatovenereology (中国皮肤性病学杂志). 2000, 14(6): 367.

[44] Wu Jin-hai, Yang Si-yuan, Jin Lan, et al. Tanshinol Influencing on Cell Adhesion Molecule Expression in Peripheral Blood Mononuclear cell (丹参素对银屑病患者外周血单个核细胞粘附分子表达的影响). *Shanghai Journal of Medical University* (上海医科大学学报). 1998, 25(1): 47.

[45] Xiao Qing-lin, Si Ben-hui, Wu Kang-zhi, et al. Variation of Hemorheology in Psoriatic Patients after Treating by Radix et Rhizoma Salviae Miltiorrhizae of Different Dosage (不同剂量丹参治疗银屑病患者后血液流变学改变). *Chinese Journal of Dermatology* (中华皮肤科杂志). 2000, 33(6): 414.

[46] Liu Bo, Li Yun-xing, Han Lei, et al. Research on Antiinflammatory and Antiimmune Action of *Yín Xiè Líng* (银屑灵抗炎及抗免疫作用的研究). *Liaoning Journal of Traditional Chinese Medicine* (辽宁中医杂志). 1999, 26(1): 37.

[47] Cheng Xue-hua, Song Yan-ping, Miao Ai-rong, et al. Pharmacological Research of *Yù Yín Piàn* (愈银片药理作用研究). *Journal of Shaanxi Traditional Chinese Medicine* (陕西中医). 1999, 20(11): 524.

[48] Gao Bing-ai, Xu Xian. Therapeutic Effect Evaluation of *Fù Fāng Shēn Dì Tāng* Matching *Dí Yín Piàn* Treating Chronic Psoriasis of Plaque Pattern (复方参地汤与迪银片联合治疗慢性斑块型银屑病的疗效评价). *Chinese Journal of Integrated Traditional and Western Medicine* (中国中西医结合杂志). 2001, 21(1): 15.

[49] Lou Wei-hai, Zhang Zhi-le, Deng Bing-rong, et al. Clinical and Experimental Study on *Liáng Xuè Huó Xuè Tāng* Treating Psoriasis in Active Stage (凉血活血汤治疗进行期银屑病的临床及实验研究). *Chinese Journal of Dermatology* (中华皮肤科杂志). 1999, 32(2): 80.

[50] Li Wei-fan, Wang Ping, Lou Wei-hai. Clinical Observation of *Liáng Xuè Huó Xuè Tāng* Treating Ordinary Psoriasis and Detection of Tumor Necrosis Factor and Interleukin-8 Levels (凉血活血汤治疗寻常型银屑病临床观察及肿瘤坏死因子和白介素 8 水平检测). *Journal of Clinical Dermatology* (临床皮肤科杂志). 2002, 31(12): 770.

[51] Yang Zhi-bo, Xiang Ya-ping, Ou-yang Heng. Comparison of Blood Serum Interleukin-6 Tumor Necrosis Factor α Levels before and after Orally Taking *Zhú Huáng Kē Lì* (银屑病患者口服竹黄颗粒剂前后血清白介素 6 和肿瘤坏死因子 α 水平的比较). *Chinese Journal of Dermatology* (中华皮肤科杂志). 2000, 33(6): 423.

[52] Luo Wen-hui, Zhang Feng-e, et al. Clinical Observation of *Zhú Huáng Kē Lì* Treating Ordinary Psoriasis (竹黄颗粒剂治疗寻常型银屑病 52 例临床观察). *Journal of Huaihua Medical College* (怀化医专学报). 2002, 1(2): 31-33.

[53] Wang Ya-juan, Shi Jing-wei, Dong Xi-lin, et al. Therapeutic Effect of *Zǐ Cǎo Huó*

Xuè Tāng Treating Psoriasis and Its Influence on Hemorheology（紫草活血汤治疗银屑病的疗效及对血液流变学的影响）. *Academic Journal of Xi'an Jiaotong University (Medical Sciences)*（西安交通大学学报，医学版）. 2003, 24(3): 275-276, 296.

[54] Song Zhi-qi, Han Shi-xin, Liu Xiao-ming, et al. Pharmacodynamic and Mechanism Research on *É Zhú Yóu Shuāng Jì* Externally Treating Psoriasis（莪术油霜剂外用治疗银屑病的药效学及作用机制研究）. *The Chinese Journal of Dermatovenereology*（中国皮肤性病学杂志）. 2001, 15(5): 301.

[55] Ma Xue-wei, Chen Guo-rong, Zhu Feng-mei, et al. Clinical Observation of *Kè Yín Yī Hào Jiāo Náng* Treating 40 Cases of Psoriasis in Active Stage（克银 I 号胶囊治疗进行期寻常型银屑病 40 例临床观察）. *Chinese Journal of Traditional Medical Science and Technology*（中医药科技）. 2000, 7(6): 396.

[56] Lin Rui-fen, Xiao Ming-hui, Wang Dou-xun. Clinical and Immunologic Research on *Sān Téng Tāng* Treating Ordinary Psoriasis（三藤汤治疗寻常型银屑病临床及免疫学研究）. *Journal of Fujian College of Traditional Chinese Medicine*（福建中医学院学报）. 2000, 10(3): 8.

[57] Feng Jie, Xu Han-qing, Su Bao-shan. *Fù Fāng Qīng Dài Jiāo Náng* Influencing on CMYC Expression in Epidermal Epithelial Cells of Psoriatic Patients（复方青黛胶囊对银屑病表皮角朊细胞中 CMYC 表达的影响）. *Chinese Journal of Integrated Traditional and Western Medicine*（中国中西医结合杂志）. 1996, 16(3): 8.

[58] Min Zhong-sheng, Wang Zi-xiong, Yang Li-jia. Clinical and Experimental Research on 71 Cases of Ordinary Psoriasis Treated by Chinese Medicinal Steaming Therapy（中药汽疗治疗寻常型银屑病 71 例临床及实验研究）. *Jiangsu Journal of Traditional Chinese Medicine*（江苏中医药）. 2002, 23(8): 12.

[59] Jiang Xiang-de, Li Jin, et al. Experimental Study on *Yín Xiè Líng Tú Mó Jì* Treating Psoriasis（银屑灵涂膜剂治疗银屑病的实验研究）. *Tianjin Journal of Traditional Chinese Medicine*（天津中医）. 2002, 19(5): 39-41.

[60] Yang Zhi-bo, Liu Zhi, et al. *Zhú Huáng Kē Lì* Influencing on Neuroendocrine Function of Psoriatic Patients in Active Stage（竹黄颗粒剂对进行期银屑病患者神经内分泌功能的影响）. *Chinese Journal of Information of Traditional Chinese Medicine*（中国中医药信息杂志）. 2002, 9(2): 15-17.

[61] Liu Ming, Qu Xing, et al. *Xiāo Yín Jiě Dú Yǐn* Influencing on Blood Serum Interleukin-8 Level in Mouse Induced by Inaurate Coccobacteria Enterotoxin of Pattern B（消银解毒饮对金黄色球菌肠毒素 B 型诱导小鼠血清白细胞介素 - 8 水平的影响）. *Chinese Journal of Integrated Traditional and Western Medicine*（中国中西医结合杂志）. 2001, 21(10): 757-759.

Cutaneous Pruritus

by **Xuan Guo-wei**, Professor & Chief Physician of Chinese External Medicine

Chi Feng-hao, Associate Chief Physician of Chinese External Medicine

Wang Lei, M.S. TCM

Huang Liang, M.S. TCM

OVERVIEW

In Chinese medicine, cutaneous pruritus belongs to the category of "Wind Itch" (*Feng Sao Yang*). Cutaneous pruritus (lit: skin itch) is a skin disease with a neurological basis. It is characterized by itchy skin that starts without actual skin damage. The cardinal symptoms are skin itchiness that manifests as a needling and burning sensation or the feeling of insects crawling on the skin. According to the area and location of pruritus, it can be classified into two categories: general pruritus and local pruritus.

Due to scratching during the course of the disease, there may be secondary signs such as hyperemia, skin damage, lichenification, hyperpigmentation, running sores or adenolymphitis (lymphadenitis). Cutaneous pruritus usually occurs in the winter and summer and is usually seen in the middle-aged and elderly. There are no fixed areas of itching and may be limited to one or two areas or it may develop extensively over the entire body. The frequency of itching is also variable, arising either intermittently or continuously and incessantly. The etiology of cutaneous pruritus is variable and can involve both internal and external factors. External factors include sudden temperature changes, skin abrasions, irritants (such as antiseptics, biocides and antibromics), dyes, and allergens (such as plants, pollens or decomposed epidermal cells). Internal factors include visceral diseases, tumors, disturbances of the nervous system, endocrine dysfunction, focal infections, diet, medications and parasites. Senile pruritus is related to the hypofunction of the glandula integumentaria.

To treat cutaneous pruritus, the etiological factors first must be determined and then followed by the avoidance of the various causative factors. Antihistamine drugs are often used to relieve itching. For general pruritus, calcium, antichlor and aethocaine are administered by intravenous injection. Adrenal cortex hormone and various kinds of antipruriginora can be applied locally.

CHINESE MEDICAL ETIOLOGY AND PATHOMECHANISM

Practitioners of traditional Chinese medicine believe both internal and external factors can be closely related to cutaneous pruritus. Internal factors are connected to disorders of the viscera (*zang-fu*), qi and blood. External factors include pathogenic wind, damp, heat and insect bites. The pathomechanism of the disease can be summarized as follows: An invasion of one of the six pathogenic factors (for example: pathogenic wind-heat or damp-heat) attacks the skin and interstitial spaces. This creates a fight with qi and blood which then moves within the interstices of the skin causes pruritus.

Due to old age and weakness, pruritus may result from Liver, Kidney and yin deficiency causing insufficient essence and blood to nourish the muscles and the skin. This causes blood dryness and the resulting wind stirring. Pruritus can also be caused by a chronic disease creating blood deficiency which generates wind due to qi and blood deficiency unable to nourish the muscles and the skin. Other causes of pruritus include the unsmooth flow of nutritive and defensive qi, meridian qi obstruction due to impairment of the seven emotions, unsmooth circulation of qi and blood from Liver qi constraint, qi stagnation and blood stasis as well as channel and vessel blockage.

Itching may be produced by an improper diet such as excessive eating of sea food or spicy and greasy food. This causes a Spleen-stomach impairment creating an intermingling of damp-heat which then transmits heat that generates wind. Itching begins when constraint in the skin and interstitial spaces is unable to drain internally (through the stool) or dispel externally (through sweating). Other causes of pruritus include Liver-gallbladder damp heat lodged in the lower *Jiao* or the retention of heat due to the blockage of dampness which then leads to malnutrition of the muscles and the skin. Unclean washing also creates pruritus when bugs and parasites multiply on the skin.

CHINESE MEDICAL TREATMENT

In using Chinese medical treatments to cure cutaneous pruritus, doctors should judge the symptoms and find an etiology based on excess or deficiency. Combined with the differentiation of signs, symptoms and diseases this will allow a thorough treatment and prevent relapse.

Pattern Differentiation and Treatment

The main principles of treating cutaneous pruritus are to eliminate pathogens to relieve itching and to regulate qi and blood.

1. Blood Heat and Hyperactivity of Pathogenic Wind

【Syndrome Characteristics】

This syndrome usually occurs in summer. Itchy skin, redness, with obvious striation. Heat easily causes itching. There may be a dry mouth and an uncalm mind. The tongue has a thin yellow coating with a red tip. The pulse is slippery and slightly rapid.

【Treatment Principle】

Clear heat to cool blood, dispel wind and relieve itching.

【Commonly Used Medicinals】

To clear heat and cool blood, use *shēng dì huáng* (Radix Rehmanniae), *dān pí* (Cortex Moutan), *chì sháo* (Radix Paeoniae Rubra). To dispel dampness, use *bái xiān pí* (Cortex Dictamni), *kǔ shēn* (Radix Sophorae Flavescentis), *huǒ má rén* (Fructus Cannabis). To dispel wind and relieve itching, use *jīng jiè* (Herba Schizonepetae), *fáng fēng* (Radix Saposhnikoviae), *chán tuì* (Periostracum Cicadae), *dì fū zǐ* (Fructus Kochiae).

【Representative Formula】

Modified *Xiāo Fēng Sǎn* (消风散).

【Ingredients】

生地黄	shēng dì huáng	15g	Radix Rehmanniae
赤芍	chì sháo	12g	Radix Paeoniae Rubra
荆芥	jīng jiè	12g	Herba Schizonepetae
防风	fáng fēng	15g	Radix Saposhnikoviae
蝉蜕	chán tuì	6g	Periostracum Cicadae
知母	zhī mǔ	15g	Rhizoma Anemarrhenae
生石膏	shēng shí gāo	15g	Gypsum Fivrosum
白鲜皮	bái xiān pí	15g	Cortex Dictamni
地肤子	dì fū zǐ	15g	Fructus Kochiae
甘草	gān cǎo	6g	Radix et Rhizoma Glycyrrhizae

Combine all the above Chinese medicinals, add 500ml of water, decoct to 100ml, and divide to take warm twice a day.

【Formula Analysis】

Jīng jiè (Herba Schizonepetae), *fáng fēng* (Radix Saposhnikoviae) and *chán tuì* (Periostracum Cicadae) are used as the chief herbs for dispersing pathogenic wind. To clear heat and cool blood therefore dispelling wind and relieving itching, use *shēng dì huáng* (Radix Rehmanniae), *chì sháo* (*Radix Paeoniae Rubra*) in combination with *bái xiān pí* (Cortex Dictamni) and *dì fū zǐ* (Fructus Kochiae) as deputies. The assistant herbs are *zhī mǔ* (Rhizoma Anemarrhenae) and *shēng shí gāo* (Gypsum Fivrosum) for clearing heat and purging pathogenic fire. For clearing heat and resolve toxinsing use *gān cǎo* (Radix et Rhizoma Glycyrrhizae) as an envoy to regulate the other herbs. The whole prescription functions to dispel wind and alleviate itching, and to clear heat and cool the blood.

【Modifications】

- If there is severe pruritus, add *wū shāo shē* (Zaocys) 15g, *cì jí lí* (Fructus Trbuli) 15g to dispel wind and relieve itching.

➢ For prolonged pruritus, add *xú cháng qīng* (Radix Cynanchi Paniculati) 12g and *mŭ dān pí* (Cortex Moutan) 15g to cool the blood, dispel wind and relieve itching.

2. Damp-heat External Invasion

【Syndrome Characteristics】

This is usually seen in the spring and summer when the weather is very hot and humid. The itching is accompanied by scattered red papules that often have yellow secretions when scratched. There is brownish urine, unsmooth defecation, a bitter taste in the mouth and agitation. The tongue is red with a yellow and greasy coating and a slippery pulse.

【Treatment Principle】

Eliminate damp to clear heat, dispel wind and relieve itching.

【Commonly Used Medicinals】

To eliminate dampness and clear heat, use *tŭ fú líng* (Rhizoma Smilacis Glabrae), *yīn chén hāo* (Herba Artemisiae Scopariae), *zé xiè* (Rhizoma Alismatis) and *yì yĭ rén* (Semen Coicis). To cool the blood and remove petechiae, use *jīn yín huā* (Flos Lonicerae), *shēng dì huáng* (Radix Rehmanniae). To dispel wind and relieve itching, use *jīng jiè* (Herba Schizonepetae), *fáng fēng* (Radix Saposhnikoviae) and *chán yī* (Periostracum).

【Representative Formula】

Tŭ Fú Líng Lì Shī Tāng (土茯苓利湿汤).

【Ingredients】

土茯苓	tŭ fú líng	20g	Rhizoma Smilacis Glabrae
茵陈蒿	yīn chén hāo	20g	Herba Artemisiae Scopariae
金银花	jīn yín huā	15g	Flos Lonicerae
生地黄	shēng dì huáng	20g	Radix Rehmanniae
泽泻	zē xiè	15g	Rhizoma Alismatis
竹叶	zhú yè	9g	Folium Bamboo

薏苡仁	yì yǐ rén	20g	Semen Coicis
防风	fáng fēng	12g	Radix Saposhnikoviae
连翘	lián qiào	12g	Fructus Forsythiae
甘草	gān cǎo	6g	Radix et Rhizoma Glycyrrhizae

Combine all the above Chinese herbs, add 500ml of water, decoct to 100ml, and divide to take warm two times.

【Formula Analysis】

Tŭ fú líng (Rhizoma Smilacis Glabrae), *jīn yín huā* (Flos Lonicerae), *yīn chén hāo* (Herba Artemisiae Scopariae) and *yì yĭ rén* (Semen Coicis) in the prescription are used as chief herbs to eliminate dampness and clear heat. *Shēng dì huáng* (Radix Rehmanniae), *zhú yè* (Folium Bamboo) and *zé xiè* (Rhizoma Alismatis) are used as deputies to clear heat and resolve toxins. For dispelling wind, clearing heat and alleviating itching, *fáng fēng* (Radix Saposhnikoviae) and *lián qiào* (Fructus Forsythiae) are used, and *gān cǎo* (Radix et Rhizoma Glycyrrhizae) is used to coordinate all the other medicinals as the Envoy.

【Modifications】

If there is pronounced itching add *dì fū zĭ* (Fructus Kochiae) 15g and *chán tuì* (Periostracum Cicadae) 10g to help eliminate damp and relieve itching.

3. Blood Deficiency and Wind Dryness

【Syndrome Characteristics】

This is often seen in older and weakened patients, or in patients with chronic diseases. It usually occurs in the autumn and winter. Symptoms include dry skin, pervasive blood spots after scratching, lusterless complexion, dizziness, and dry stool. The tongue is pink with a white thin coating and a thready pulse.

【Treatment Principle】

Moisten dryness by enriching blood, dispel wind to relieve itching.

【Commonly Used Medicinals】

To moisten dryness by enriching blood, use *dāng guī* (Radix Angelicae Sinensis), *shēng dì huáng* (Radix Rehmanniae Recens), *bái sháo* (Raidix Paeoniae Alba), *chuān xiōng* (Rhizoma Chuanxiong) and *hé shǒu wū* (Radix Polygoni Multiflori) are used. To dispel wind and relieve itching use *jīng jiè* (Herba Schizonepetae) and *cì jí lí* (Fructus Trbuli). To tonify yin and moisten dryness use *mài mén dōng* (Raidix Ophiopogonis) and *yù zhú* (Rhizoma Polygonati Odorati).

【Representative Formula】

Modified *Dāng Guī Yǐn Zi* (当归饮子).

【Ingredients】

当归	dāng guī	9g	Radix Angelicae Sinensis
生地黄	shēng dì huáng	15g	Radix Rehmanniae Recens
白芍	bái sháo	9g	Raidix Paeoniae Alba
川芎	chuān xiōng	3g	Rhizoma Chuanxiong
何首乌	hé shǒu wū	15g	Radix Polygoni Multiflori
荆芥	jīng jiè	6g	Herba Schizonepetae
刺蒺藜	cì jí lí	9g	Fructus Trbuli
防风	fáng fēng	9g	Radix Saposhnikoviae
麦门冬	mài mén dōng	15g	Raidix Ophiopogonis
玉竹	yù zhú	15g	Rhizoma Polygonati Odorati
甘草	gān cǎo	6g	Radix et Rhizoma Glycyrrhizae

Combine the above Chinese medicinals, add 500ml of water, decoct to 100ml, take warm twice a day.

【Formula Analysis】

Dāng guī (Radix Angelicae Sinensis), *bái sháo* (Raidix Paeoniae Alba), *chuān xiōng* (Rhizoma Chuanxiong), *hé shǒu wū* (Radix Polygoni Multiflori) and *shēng dì huáng* (Radix Rehmanniae) are used to enrich the blood and moisten the skin as chief herbs. *Mài mén dōng* (Raidix Ophiopogonis) and *yù zhú* (Rhizoma Polygonati Odorati) are used to enrich yin and moisten dryness as deputies. *Jīng jiè* (Herba Schizonepetae), *cì jí lí*

(Fructus Trbuli) and *fáng fēng* (Radix Saposhnikoviae) dispel wind and relieve itching (assistants). *Gān cǎo* (Radix et Rhizoma Glycyrrhizae) is used to harmonize the other herbs (envoy). The whole prescription primarily functions to enrich yin essence and nourish blood while giving consideration to dispelling wind and alleviating itching. This treats both the symptoms and the root of the disease.

【Modifications】

➢ If there is extreme itching, add *quán xiē* (Scorpio) 6g and *wū shāo shé* (Zaocys) 15g to expel exterior and interior wind.

➢ If there is prolonged pruritus, dark purple erythema, purplish tongue with stasis spots and rough pulse, add *dān shēn* (Radix Salviae Miltiorrhiae) 20g to invigorate blood and transform stasis to relieve itching.

➢ When there is irritability and reduced sleep, subtract *chuān xiōng* (Rhizoma Chuanxiong) and add *bǎi zǐ rén* (Semen Platycladi) 15g, *yuǎn zhì* (Radix Polygalae) 10g and *mǔ dān pí* (Cortex Moutan) 15g to clear deficient fire, nourish Heart and calm the mind. For dry stool constipation add *bǎi zǐ rén* (Semen Platycladi) 15g and *huǒ má rén* (Semen Cannabis).

4. Yin Deficiency and Hyperactivity of Wind

【Syndrome Characteristics】

Obstinate and protracted itching all over the body, deepening of the dermal ridge and lichenoid skin. Red or crimson and dry tongue, without coating, wiry and thready or rapid pulse.

【Treatment Principle】

Enrich yin essence and clear heat, dispel wind to relieve itching.

【Commonly Used Medicinals】

To enrich yin essence and clear heat use *shēng dì huáng* (Radix Rehmanniae), *mài mén dōng* (Raidix Ophiopogonis), *xuán shēn* (Raidix

Scrophulariae)and *bái sháo* (Raidix Paeoniae Alba). To dispel wind and relieve itching, use *jīng jiè* (Herba Schizonepetae), *fáng fēng* (Radix Saposhnikoviae) and *wū shāo shé* (Zaocys).

【Representative Formula】

Modified *Yǎng Yīn Qīng Fèi Tāng* (养阴清肺汤).

【Ingredients】

生地黄	shēng dì huáng	30g	Radix Rehmanniae Recens
麦门冬	mài mén dōng	15g	Raidix Ophiopogonis
玄参	xuán shēn	15g	Raidix Scrophulariae
牡丹皮	mǔ dān pí	9g	Cortex Moutan
白芍	bái sháo	9g	Raidix Paeoniae Alba
荆芥	jīng jiè	6g	Herba Schizonepetae
防风	fáng fēng	9g	Radix Saposhnikoviae
蜈蚣	wú gōng	2 strips	Scolopendra
乌梢蛇	wū shāo shē	15g	Zaocys
甘草	gān cǎo	6g	Radix et Rhizoma Glycyrrhizae

Put the above Chinese medicinals in 500ml of water and decoct down to 100ml. Take warm twice a day.

【Formula Analysis】

Mài mén dōng (Raidix Ophiopogonis), *xuán shēn* (Raidix Scrophulariae) and *bái sháo* (Raidix Paeoniae Alba) are used as chief herbs to nourish yin and clear heat. The deputies, *jīng jiè* (Herba Schizonepetae), *fáng fēng* (Radix Saposhnikoviae), *wú gōng* (Scolopendra) and *wū shāo shé* (Zaocys) dispel wind and remove obstructions in the meridians. This will relieve itching. *Shēng dì huáng* (Radix Rehmanniae) and *mǔ dān pí* (Cortex Moutan) are used as assistants to clear heat and cool blood. *Gān cǎo* (Radix et Rhizoma Glycyrrhizae) is used to harmonize the other herbs as the envoy.

【Modifications】

- For dry skin and desquamation add *jī xuè téng* (Caulis Spatholobi)

30g and *shān zhū yú* (Fructus Corni) 9g to tonify blood and yin and relieve itching.

➤ For a dry mouth and lips add *pí pá yè* (Folium Eriobtryae) 15g , *yù zhú* (Rhizoma Polygonati Odorati) 15g and *shí hú* (Herba Dendrobii) 15g in order to nourish yin and moisten dryness.

➤ If there are symptoms such as somasthenia (chronic physical fatigue) and hypodynamia (diminished strength), dry mouth and thirst, thready and weak pulse, it is considered as a syndrome of qi and yin deficiency. Therefore take out *mǔ dān pí* (Cortex Moutan) and add *tài zǐ shēn* (Radix Pseudostellariae) 15g to invigorate the Spleen and replenish qi.

➤ For indigestion, lack of appetite and oral blandness add *bái zhú* (Rhizoma Atractylodis Macrocephalae) 15g and *fú líng* (Poria) 30g to invigorate the Spleen to transform damp.

5. Blood Stasis

【Syndrome Characteristics】

Itchy skin which is worse at night, aggravated when exposed to cold or heat, widespread striation, purplish skin or with nodus. Purple tongue, usually rough pulse.

【Treatment Principle】

Regulate the flow of qi and invigorate blood.

【Commonly Used Medicinals】

To regulate the flow of qi and invigorate blood use *dāng guī* (Radix Angelicae Sinensis), *táo rén* (Semen Persicae), *hóng huā* (Flos Carthami) and *chì sháo* (Radix Paeoniae Rubra). To expel wind and to relieve itching, use *jīng jiè* (Herba Schizonepetae), *cì jí lí* (Fructus Trbuli) and *chán tuì* (Periostracum Cicadae).

【Representative Formula】

Modified *Huó Xuè Qū Fēng Tāng* (活血祛风汤).

【Ingredients】

当归	dāng guī	9g	Radix Angelicae Sinensis
桃仁	táo rén	9g	Semen Persicae
红花	hóng huā	6g	Flos Carthami
赤芍	chì sháo	9g	Radix Paeoniae Rubra
荆芥	jīng jiè	9g	Herba Schizonepetae
刺蒺藜	cì jí lí	15g	Fructus Trbuli
蝉蜕	chán tuì	6g	Periostracum Cicadae
防风	fáng fēng	9g	Radix Saposhnikoviae
枳壳	zhǐ qiào	15g	Fructus Aurantii
茯苓	fú líng	15g	Poria
甘草	gān cǎo	3g	Radix et Rhizoma Glycyrrhizae

Combine all the above Chinese medicinals, add 500ml water, decoct to 100ml, and divide to take warm two times.

【Formula Analysis】

The prescription uses *dāng guī* (Radix Angelicae Sinensis), *táo rén* (Semen Persicae) and *hóng huā* (Flos Carthami) for invigorating blood and transforming stasis as the chief herbs. It uses *chì sháo* (Radix Paeoniae Rubra) and *zhǐ qiào* (Fructus Aurantii) for regulating the flow of qi and transforming stasis and *jīng jiè* (Herba Schizonepetae), *cì jí lí* (Fructus Trbuli), *chán tuì* (Periostracum Cicadae) and *fáng fēng* (Radix Saposhnikoviae) for expelling wind to relieve itching. All are deputies. It uses the assistants, *fú líng* (Poria) to invigorate the Spleen and calm the mind. *Gān cǎo* (Radix et Rhizoma Glycyrrhizae) is used to coordinate the other medicinals as the envoy.

【Modifications】

➢ If there are heat signs, add *xuán shēn* (Raidix Scrophulariae) 15g, *zhī zǐ* (Fructus Gardeniae) 15g to clear heat and resolve toxins. For itching in the lower part of the body, add *dì lóng* (Pheretima) 12g, *niú xī* (Radix Acanthopanacis Bidentatae) 15g to extinguish wind and invigorate stasis and regulate the flow of qi to relieve itching.

➢ For itching with fluctuating emotions add *gōu téng* (Ramulus Uncariae Cum Uncis) 10g, *shí jué míng* (Concha Haliotidis) 30g and *chuān liàn zǐ* (Fuctus Toosendan) 9g to calm the Liver and extinguish wind and relieve itching by regulating the flow of qi.

Additional Treatment Modalities

1. Chinese patent Medicine

1) *Wū Shé Zhǐ Yǎng Wán* (乌蛇止痒丸)

3-5g, 2 times a day. It is suitable for pruritus with blood deficiency and a dry wind pattern.

2) *Shī Dú Qīng* (湿毒清)

3 capsules, 3 times a day. It is suitable for pruritus with a damp-heat pattern.

3) *Liù Wèi Dì Huáng Wán* (六味地黄丸)

5g, 2 times a day. It is used for pruritus for older people and/or persons with a yin deficiency pattern.

2. Acupuncture and Moxibustion

(1) Body Acupuncture Therapy

【Point Selection】

LI 11	qū chí	曲池
ST 36	zú sān lǐ	足三里
SP 6	sān yīn jiāo	三阴交
SP 10	xuè hǎi	血海

【Point Modifications】

➢ For pruritus vulvae, add SP 9 (*yīn líng quán*) and BL23 (*shèn shù*).

➢ For pruritus of the anus add DU 1 (*cháng qiáng*), RN 3 (*zhōng jí*), and BL 57 (*chéng shān*).

➢ For pruritus on the scalp add GB 20 (*fēng chí*).

【Manipulation】

For excess syndrome use the reducing method, while for deficiency syndrome, use the reinforcing method. After obtaining qi, retain the needle for 30 minutes, once a day, ten times as a course of therapy.

(2) Auriculotherapy

【Point Selection】

shenmen	TF4	神门
adrenal gland	TG2	肾上腺
Itching points		

【Manipulation】

Insert the needle quickly, retain for 30 minutes, once a day. This method of needling can also be used once a week.

(3) Moxibustion

【Point Selection】

Use corresponding points in the areas of itching.

【Manipulation】

Choose corresponding points, use burning moxa sticks held over the points, 20min each time, 1-2 times a day, ten days as a course. For older patients, RN 8 (*shén quē*) could be used. For pruritus ani, use DU 1 (*cháng qiáng*) for moxibustion.

(4) Posterior Blood-letting Therapy

【Manipulation】

Sterilize the posterior surface of the ear. Puncture the vein in back of the ear with a sterilized three-edged needling, and release a few spots of blood until it stops on its own. Do this once a week.

(5) Scalp Acupuncture

【Manipulation】

At the upper 2/5 part of the sensory region and foot region bilaterally, insert the needle quickly, rotate skillfully for about 1 minute, retain for 30 minutes, once a day.

(6) External Treatment

1) Chinese Medicinal Lotion

a)

荆芥	jīng jiè	30g	Herba Schizonepetae
黄精	huáng jīng	30g	Rhizoma Polygonati
蛇床子	shé chuáng zǐ	30g	Fructus Cnidii
川芎	chuān xiōng	20g	Rhizoma Chuanxiong
赤芍	chì sháo	20g	Radix Paeoniae Rubra
苦参	kǔ shēn	30g	Radix Sophorae Flavescentis
野菊花	yě jú huā	30g	Flos Chrysanthemi Indici

Combine the above Chinese herbs and simmer in 2000ml of water to use as a warm external skin wash. Suitable for pruritus with a blood deficiency and dry wind pattern.

b)

苦参	kǔ shēn	30g	Radix Sophorae Flavescentis
蛇床子	shé chuáng zǐ	30g	Fructus Cnidii
苍耳子	cāng ěr zǐ	30g	Fructus Xanthii
艾叶	ài yè	15g	Folium Artemisiae Argyi

Decoct in water and use the decoction for an external wash.

2) Liniment

a) *Qū Fēng Zhǐ Yǎng Shuāng* (祛风止痒霜)

荆芥	jīng jiè	15g	Herba Schizonepetae
防风	fáng fēng	15g	Radix Saposhnikoviae
蛇床子	shé chuáng zǐ	15g	Fructus Cnidii
徐长卿	xú cháng qīng	15g	Radix Cynanchi Paniculati
乌梅	wū méi	20g	Fructus Mume

苦参	kǔ shēn	20g	Radix Sophorae Flavescentis
冰片	bīng piàn	5g	Broneolum Syntheticum
薄荷脑	bò hé nǎo	3g	Mentholum

All of the above Chinese medicinals are made into a cream and applied to the affected parts twice a day.

b) Calamine lotion for external use.

3. Simple Prescriptions and Empirical Formulas

(1) Use equal amounts of *kǔ shēn* (Radix Sophorae Flavescentis) and *xú cháng qīng* (Radix Cynanchi Paniculati), grind into fine powder and make into tablets, each tablet weighing 0.5g. Take 3-5 tablets 3 times a day.

(2) With equal amounts of *fú píng* (Herba Spirodelae) and *cāng ěr zǐ* (Fructus Xanthii), grind into a powder and make them into honey pills with each pill weighing 9g. Take one pill in both the morning and night.

(3) Grind *chán tuì* (Periostracum Cicadae) 30g into a fine powder, 1g, 2 times a day.

(4) *Bái xiān pí* (Cortex Dictamni) 30g, *cì jí lí* (Fructus Trbuli) 30g and *cāng ěr zǐ* (Fructus Xanthii) 30g, decoct into a warm external wash to be used twice a day.

(5) *Wǔ wèi zǐ* (Fructus Schisandrae) 30g, *jiāo mù* (Semen Zanthoxyli) 10g, decocted into a warm external wash, twice a day.

(6) *Cì jí lí* (Fructus Trbuli) 20g and *zào jiǎo cì* (Spina Gleditsiae) 30g are decocted into a warm external wash to be used once a day.

(7) *Huáng bǎi* (Cortex Phellodendri) 30g, decoct to wash, once a day.

PROGNOSIS

After the symptomatic treatment of pruritus to eliminate etiological factors, symptoms can quickly disappear. Because of repeated scratching, obstinate pruritus due to the dysfunction of the internal organs may lead to lichenification of the skin and hyperpigmentation. Scratched skin can easily become infected and complicated by pyoderma (skin purulence) and adenolymphitis (lymph inflammation). Itching can also cause sleep disturbance or "neurasthenia". For pruritus caused by an internal malignant tumor, especially severe itching indicates an unfavorable prognosis and an acceleration of the worsening of the disease.

PREVENTIVE HEALTHCARE

There are various complicated internal and external etiological factors which can cause pruritus. Consequently one must be careful to avoid those conditions that can provoke a relapse. Special attention should be paid to regulate the diet and to protect the skin. For this reason attention should be paid to the following points:

Lifestyle Modification

(1) Take note of climactic influences and avoid attacks of cold wind and bedding that is too warm. In the summertime avoid the stimulation of sweat. Promptly change clothes corresponding to changes of climate to reduce skin irritation.

(2) Avoid contact or inhalation of environmental substances such as lacquer paints, pollens, cosmetics and dust mites. Maintain the indoor air clean and fresh. Pay attention to skin hygiene. Do not use alkaline cleaning soap or solutions. The use of mild cleaning agents is recommended. Avoid bathing too often, especially in winter. Washing in very hot water should be avoided. For pruritus ani and pruritus vulvae, wash with warm, clean water rather than soap after defecation. 100 percent cotton fabrics are most suitable for underwear and should be loose and comfortable. Do not wear rubber or plastic shoes or nylon stockings.

Dietary Recommendation

It is better to eat mild flavored food, such as vegetables and fruits. Avoid smoking, alcohol, strong teas, coffee and eating spicy food. Most of the diet should be of green vegetables and fruits. Maintain regular bowel movements.

Regulation of Emotional and Mental Health

Keep a stable and calm emotional life. Sleep at the right time and lead an orderly life. Be optimistic when facing problems. (Make patients aware of the harmfulness of scratching, and tell them to try to maintain control and restraint when there is the temptation to scratch.)

CLINICAL EXPERIENCE OF RENOWNED PHYSICIANS

Empirical Formulas

1. *Quán Chóng Fāng* (全虫方) for Curing Stubborn Pruritus (Zhao Bing-nan)

【Syndrome Characteristics】

Prolonged itching of skin, rough skin, with obvious striation and blood crusts but no effusion of fluids. Suitable for chronic pruritus characterized by an excess syndrome.

【Ingredients】

全虫	quán chóng	6g	Scorpio
皂角刺	zào jiǎo cì	12g	Spina Gleditsiae
猪牙皂角	zhū yá zào jiǎo	6g	Fructus Gleditsiae Abnormalis
刺蒺藜	cì jí lí	15-30g	Fructus Trbuli
炒槐花	chǎo huái huā	15-30g	Flos Sophorae Praeparata Tostum
威灵仙	wēi líng xiān	12-30g	Radix et Rhizoma Clematidis
苦参	kǔ shēn	6g	Radix Sophorae Flavescentis
白鲜皮	bái xiān pí	15g	Cortex Dictamni
黄柏	huáng bǎi	15g	Cortex Phellodendri Chinensis

Combine the above Chinese medicinals, add 500 ml of water, decoct to 100ml and divide to take warm twice a day.

【Formula analysis】

Quán chóng (Scorpio), *zào jiāo cì* (Spina Gleditsiae) and *zhū yá zào* (Fructus Gleditsiae Abnormalis) are used as chief herbs in the prescription. *Quán chóng* (Scorpio), is pungent in flavor and neutral in property and enters the Liver meridian. It has a mobilizing and opening nature and is able to extinguish exterior and interior pathogenic wind. *Zào jiāo cì* (Spina Gleditsiae) is pungent in flavor and warm in property and functions to dispel toxic swelling and draw out pus. It also eliminates pathogenic wind and kills parasites. *Zhū yá zào* (Fructus Gleditsiae Abnormalis) can clear the qi of the Lung and Large Intestine, clears stagnant dampness in the Stomach and Intestine and functions to dissipate pathogenic wind, alleviate itching and resolve toxins.

The nature of heat is to scatter, while damp toxins tend to gather. If the intent is to remove damp toxins one must apply both attacking and dissipating methods. The above three Chinese medicinals are used together to extinguish wind, alleviate itching and resolve toxins. This makes them suitable for obstinate and prolonged pruritus due to dampness.

Bái xiān pí (Cortex Dictamni) is cold in property, bitter in flavor and dry in nature. It is able to clear heat, dispel wind, eliminate dampness and alleviate itching. Together with *kǔ shēn* (Radix Sophorae Flavescentis) it assists *quán chóng* (Scorpio) to dispel superficial exterior wind and damp accumulation to alleviate itching. *Cì jí lí* (Fructus Trbuli) is warm and bitter and dispels wind, *"curing various wind skin diseases" and "wind-itching in the body"*. It is good at relieving itching. Together with *wēi líng xiān* (Radix et Rhizoma Clematidis) it assists *quán chóng* (Scorpio) to remove pathogenic wind and accumulated dampness deep in the body.

In addition, the stagnation of qi in the Spleen and Stomach results in the retention of dampness. This generates toxicity and obstinate damp toxins that causes endless itching on the skin. Therefore, *chǎo zhǐ qiào* (Fructus Aurantii Tostum), *chǎo huái huā* (Flos Sophorae Tostum) and *huáng bǎi* (Cortex Phellodendri Chinensis) are used as envoys to promote qi circulation, and clear binding heat in the stomach and intestines. These are directed towards regulating the function of the stomach and intestines and removing the source of accumulated damp-heat. By addressing both the root and branch, deeper levels of cure can be reached.

【Modifications】

- If the prescription does not take effect, add *wū shāo shé* (Zaocys) 10g.
- For severe itching, with damage to the skin, obvious hyperpigmentation or accompanied by dry stool add *dà huáng* (Radix et Rhizoma Rhei) 9-15g.

(Mi Yi'e: Editor-in-chief. *Selected Effective Secret Recipe from Famous Physicians of Chinese Medicine of the First National Grade* (*Sequel*). 首批国家级名老中医效验秘方精选(续集). Beijing: China Today Publishing House 今日中国出版社, 1999: 423-424)

2. *Pí Xuǎn Tāng* (皮癣汤) for Curing Pruritus of Heat Syndrome (Zhu Ren-kang)

【Syndrome Characteristics】

Generalized neurodermatitis, cutaneous pruritus, eczema with papule eruption. Manifested by flaky small red papule, severe itching, red tongue with white thin coating, wiry and slippery pulse.

【Treatment Principle】

Cool blood and clear heat, eliminate wind to relieve itching.

【Ingredients】

生地黄	shēng dì huáng	30g	Radix Rehmanniae Recens
牡丹皮	mǔ dān pí	9g	Cortex Moutan
赤芍	chì sháo	9g	Radix Paeoniae Rubra
苍耳子	cāng ěr zǐ	9g	Fructus Xanthii

白鲜皮	bái xiān pí	9g	Cortex Dictamni
苦参	kŭ shēn	9g	Radix Sophorae Flavescentis
地肤子	dì fū zĭ	9g	Fructus Kochiae
黄芩	huáng qín	9g	Radix Scutellariae
生甘草	shēng gān căo	9g	Radix et Rhizoma Glycyrrhizae (raw)

Combine the above Chinese medicinals, add 500 ml of water, decoct to 100ml, and divide to take warm twice a day.

【Formula analysis】

To cool blood and moisten dryness, use *shēng dì huáng* (Radix Rehmanniae Recens), *dāng guī* (Radix Angelicae Sinensis) and *chì sháo* (Radix Paeoniae Rubra). To clear heat and resolve toxins, use *huáng qín* (Radix Scutellariae) and *gān căo* (Radix et Rhizoma Glycyrrhizae). To expel wind and remove dampness, clear heat and relieve itching, use *cāng ĕr zĭ* (Fructus Xanthii), *kŭ shēn* (Radix Sophorae Flavescentis), *bái xiān pí* (Cortex Dictamni) and *dì fū zĭ* (Fructus Kochiae).

(Mi Yi'e: Editor-in-chief. *Selected Effective Secret Recipe from Famous Physicians of Chinese Medicine of the First National Grade* (*Sequel*). 首批国家级名老中医效验秘方精选 (续集). Beijing: China Today Publishing House 今日中国出版社 , 1999: 422)

Selected Case Studies

1. Case Studies of Zhu Ren-kang—Blood Deficiency and Wind Hyperactivity

【Initial Visit】

Ms. Liao, age 72. First visit: September 21st 1974.

Chief complaint: Severe itching all over the body for four months, worsening at night, less sleep at night.

She was already taking prescriptions with the actions of cooling blood and clearing heat, expelling wind and removing damp, yet there was no relief. Dry stool or sometimes had difficulty in defecation, once every five days.

Examination: Dry and loose skin, visible striation, with fine and thin squamae, widespread blood crusts. Wiry and slippery pulse, purple tongue with bare coating.

【Pattern Differentiation】

Blood deficiency and impairment of yin, unable to nourish the skin due to old age, hyperactivity of wind causing dryness, and hyperactivity of wind causing itching.

【Treatment Principle】

Enrich blood and moisten dryness, invigorate blood and expel wind.

【Ingredients】

当归	dāng guī	12g	Radix Angelicae Sinensis
白芍	bái sháo	9g	Radix Paeoniae Alba
熟地黄	shú dì huáng	30g	Radix Rehmanniae Praeparata
玄参	xuán shēn	9g	Radix Scrophulariae
麦门冬	mài mén dōng	9g	Radix Ophiopogonis
牡丹皮	mǔ dān pí	9g	Cortex Moutan
红花	hóng huā	9g	Flos Carthami
荆芥	jīng jiè	9g	Herba Schizonepetae
刺蒺藜	cì jí lí	9g	Fructus Trbuli
火麻仁	huǒ má rén	9g	Fructus Cannabis
甘草	gān cǎo	6g	Radix et Rhizoma Glycyrrhizae

Six packets, decoct in water.

【Second Visit】

Second visit: October 31st 1974. The symptoms of itching dramatically improved after medication. She was able to sleep at night. Wiry pulse, crimson tongue without coating.

【Third Visit】

Third visit: November 16th 1974. After medication the symptoms of itching had been alleviated greatly. However in the last few days the itching was again severe with small red pimples after scratching. Dry stool. Wiry and thready pulse, purple tongue with bare coating, thin and yellow in the center.

【Ingredients】

当归	dāng guī	12g	Radix Angelicae Sinensis
赤芍	chì sháo	9g	Radix Paeoniae Rubra
桃仁	táo rén	9g	Semen Persicae
红花	hóng huā	9g	Flos Carthami
玄参	xuán shēn	9g	Radix Scrophulariae
荆芥	jīng jiè	9g	Herba Schizonepetae
刺蒺藜	cì jí lí	9g	Fructus Trbuli
牡丹皮	mŭ dān pí	9g	Cortex Moutan
火麻仁	huŏ má rén	9g	Fructus Cannabis
甘草	gān căo	6g	Radix et Rhizoma Glycyrrhizae

Six packets.

【Fourth Visit】

Fourth visit: January 9th 1975. The itching became lighter but was still felt in the breast, abdomen, waistline and back of the body. Wiry pulse, bare and peeled tongue, thin and yellow coat in the center. Instruct the patient to continue to take the prescription of the initial visit, six packets. Following up with the patient in May, 1975, the patient had fully recovered.

(Edited by Guang An Men Hospital of Academy Institute of Chinese Medicine. *Clinical Experience Collection of Zhu Ren-kang* 朱仁康临床经验集. People's Medical Publishing House 人民卫生出版社, 1979: 138)

2. Case Studies of Zhang Zhi-li—Retention Wind and Heat of Skin

【Initial Visit】

Mr Sheng, age 50. Initial visit: July 5th 1989.

Chief Complaint: After using a hair dye 8 months ago, it created an allergic reaction. After treatment the swelling vanished, but still suffered from paroxysmal itching on the skin of the face, especially after drinking. Restless, relieved a little after scratching until bleeding and painful. Worsening due to seasonal sweating on dry and hot summer days. Recently symptoms of itching over the whole body had developed, influencing his sleep. In the daytime there was dizziness and fatigue. Bitter taste in the mouth, poor digestion and appetite, the pain and suffering were becoming unbearable.

Examination: Itching over the entire body, widespread striation, striping on the surface and blood crusts scattered on the surface. Some lichenification, some parts of skin with some papula around the hair follicles, rough skin. Red tongue tip, white and greasy coating, wiry and slightly rapid pulse.

【Pattern Differentiation】

Retention of wind-damp, unable to nourish skin.

【Treatment Principle】

Expel wind and remove dampness, enrich blood and moisten skin.

【Ingredients】

全虫	quán chóng	6g	Scorpio
皂角刺	zào jiăo cì	6g	Spina Gleditsiae
刺蒺藜	cì jí lí	30g	Fructus Trbuli
白鲜皮	bái xiān pí	30g	Cortex Dictamni
苦参	kŭ shēn	15g	Radix Sophorae Flavescentis
车前子	chē qián zĭ	15g	Semen Plantaginis
车前草	chē qián căo	15g	Herba Plantaginis
泽泻	zé xiè	10g	Rhizoma Alismatis
生白术	shēng bái zhú	10g	Rhizoma Atractylodis Macrocephalae (raw)
生枳壳	shēng zhĭ qiào	10g	Fructus Aurantii (raw)
生地黄	shēng dì huáng	15g	Radix Rehmanniae Recens
生槐花	shēng huái huā	30g	Flos Sophorae (raw)
当归	dāng guī	10g	Radix Angelicae Sinensis
夜交藤	yè jiāo téng	30g	Caulis Polygoni Multiflori

地肤子	dì fū zǐ	15g	Fructus Kochiae
防风	fáng fēng	10g	Radix Saposhnikoviae

External use: Decoct *mǎ chǐ xiàn* (Herba Portulaca) 30g in water. After cooling take the decoction to wash the affected parts, then add 15g of *Xióng Huáng Jiě Dú Sǎn* (雄黄解毒散) (Realgar Powder for Detoxication) in 60ml of *Bǎi Bù Jiǔ* (百部酒), shake to mix them together for external use.

【Second Visit】

After treatment for 2 weeks the itching symptoms were much relieved and she slept for about 6 hours during the night and her spirit and appetite also improved. So subtract *quán chóng* (Scorpio), *chē qián cǎo* (Herba Plantaginis) and *shēng huái huā* (Flos Sophorae) from the former prescription, and add *dān shēn* (Radix et Rhizoma Salviae Miltiorrhizae) 15g, *jī xuè téng* (Caulis Spatholobi) 30g and *chì sháo* (Radix Paeoniae Rubra) 15g.

【Third Visit】

After taking another 14 packets the symptoms of itching vanished. Under examination, except for incomplete regression of lichenification, there was no visible striation nor blood scabs. Continue to take medicine for maintenance with 5% *Hēi Dòu Liú Yóu Ruǎn Gāo* (黑豆馏油软膏) for external use.

(Edited by An Jia-feng and Zhang Fan. *Selected Zhang Zhi-li Medical Cases of Dermatogic Disease* 张志礼皮肤病医案选萃. People's Medical Publishing House 人民卫生出版社, 1994: 155)

Discussions

1. Zhu Ren-kang's Principles of Treating Wind

There are many factors causing cutaneous pruritus, but there is always pathogenic wind, from either external or internal wind. External wind involves wind-heat, wind-damp, while internal wind involves blood heat generating wind, blood deficiency generating wind and blood stasis generating wind. Blood heat generating wind is usually seen in summer pruritus and in the prime of the patient's life. Blood deficiency generating wind is often seen among older people and in winter. Pattern differentiation is as follows:

1) Blood Heat

Blood heat generating wind due to Heart fire. This manifests as itching of the skin, redness, scratching creates bleeding, easy to feel itchy with heat, or with a dry mouth and agitation. It usually occurs in the summer. Wiry and slippery with rapid pulse, crimson tongue or red tongue tip, yellow thin coating. Principles: cool blood to clear heat, expel wind to relieve itching. Formula: Modified *Zhǐ Yǎng Xī Fēng Tāng* (止痒熄风汤).

【Ingredients】

生地黄	shēng dì huáng	30g	Radix Rehmanniae Recens
牡丹皮	mŭ dān pí	9g	Cortex Moutan
赤芍	chì sháo	9g	Radix Paeoniae Rubra
丹参	dān shēn	9g	Radix et Rhizoma Salviae Miltiorrhizae
玄参	xuán shēn	9g	Radix Scrophulariae
白鲜皮	bái xiān pí	9g	Cortex Dictamni
煅龙骨	duàn lóng gŭ	10g	Os Draconis Praeparata
煅牡蛎	duàn mŭ lì	10g	Concha Ostreae Praeparata
刺蒺藜	cì jí lí	9g	Fructus Trbuli
生甘草	shēng gān căo	6g	Radix et Rhizoma Glycyrrhizae (raw)

2) Blood Deficiency

This is usually seen in pruritus senilis and occurs in the autumn and winter. It is caused by both qi and blood deficiency, when the blood can not nourish the skin and Liver-wind is generated from the interior. The hyperactivity of pathogenic wind creates the pruritus. The symptoms are dry skin, widespread scattered scratch marks, lusterless complexion or dizziness, palpitations, nervousness and insomnia. Wiry and thready pulse, light tongue with clean coating. Principle: To enrich blood and moisten dryness, dissipate wind to relieve itching. Formula: Modified *Dāng Guī Yǐn Zi* (当归饮子) or *Yǎng Xuè Rùn Fū Yǐn* (养血润肤饮).

【Ingredients】

生地	shēng dì	12g	Radix Rehmanniae Recens
熟地	shú dì	12g	Prepared Radix Rehmanniae Praeparata
何首乌	hé shǒu wū	12g	Radix Polygoni Multiflori
当归	dāng guī	9g	Radix Angelicae Sinensis
白芍	bái sháo	9g	Radix Paeoniae Alba
荆芥	jīng jiè	9g	Herba Schizonepetae
刺蒺藜	cì jí lí	9g	Fructus Trbuli
黄芪	huáng qí	12g	Radix Astragali
火麻仁	huǒ má rén	9g	Fructus Cannabis
麦门冬	mài mén dōng	9g	Radix Ophiopogonis
甘草	gān cǎo	9g	Radix et Rhizoma Glycyrrhizae

3) Wind-Damp

It is caused by internal Spleen-stomach damp-heat retention with an attack by external pathogenic wind. Manifestations include itchy skin where scratching brings watery blisters, bloody rashes or changing into something like eczema. Wiry and slippery pulse, white greasy or white thin and greasy tongue fur. Principle: expel wind and eliminate dampness, clear heat and relieve itching. Formula: Modified *Xiāo Fēng Sǎn* (消风散).

【Ingredients】

荆芥	jīng jiè	9g	Herba Schizonepetae
防风	fáng fēng	6g	Radix Saposhnikoviae
羌活	qiāng huó	9g	Rhizoma et Radix Notopterygii
蝉蜕	chán tuì	4.5g	Periostracum Cicadae
陈皮	chén pí	6g	Pericarpium Citri Reticulatae

茯苓	fú líng	9g	Poria
白芷	bái zhǐ	4.5g	Radix Angelicae Dahuricae
枳壳	zhǐ qiào	9g	Fructus Aurantii
金银花	jīn yín huā	9g	Flos Lonicerae Japonicae
甘草	gān cǎo	6g	Radix et Rhizoma Glycyrrhizae

4) Heavy Wind

"Heavy Wind (*Zhong Feng*)" refers to a prolonged retention of pathogenic wind that has transformed into heat and dryness. Manifestations are obstinate, protracted and include itching over the entire body and lichenification. The pulse is wiry and thready and there is a red tongue with yellow thin coating. The Treatment principle is to remove wind and purge heat. Formula: *Wū Shé Qū Fēng Tāng* (乌蛇驱风汤).

【Ingredients】

乌梢蛇	wū shāo shé	9g	Zaocys
蝉蜕	chán tuì	6g	Periostracum Cicadae
荆芥	jīng jiè	9g	Herba Schizonepetae
防风	fáng fēng	9g	Radix Saposhnikoviae
羌活	qiāng huó	9g	Rhizoma et Radix Notopterygii
白芷	bái zhǐ	6g	Radix Angelicae Dahuricae
黄连	huáng lián	6g	Rhizoma Coptidis
黄芩	huáng qín	9g	Radix Scutellariae
金银花	jīn yín huā	9g	Flos Lonicerae Japonicae
连翘	lián qiào	9g	Fructus Forsythiae
甘草	gān cǎo	6g	Radix et Rhizoma Glycyrrhizae

5) Pruritus Scroti

Zī Yīn Chú Shī Tāng (滋阴除湿汤).

【Ingredients】

生地黄	shēng dì huáng	30g	Radix Rehmanniae Recens
玄参	xuán shēn	12g	Radix Scrophulariae

当归	dāng guī	12g	Radix Angelicae Sinensis
丹参	dān shēn	15g	Radix et Rhizoma Salviae Miltiorrhizae
茯苓	fú líng	9g	Poria
泽泻	zé xiè	9g	Rhizoma Alismatis
白鲜皮	bái xiān pí	9g	Cortex Dictamni
蛇床子	shé chuáng zǐ	9g	Fructus Cnidii
煅龙骨	duàn lóng gǔ	15g	Os Draconis Praeparata
煅牡蛎	duàn mǔ lì	15g	Concha Ostreae Praeparata

Xī xiān cǎo (Herba Siegesbeckiae), *kǔ shēn* (Radix Sophorae Flavescentis), *dì fū zǐ* (Fructus Kochiae) and *bái xiān pí* (Cortex Dictamni) are decocted, apply the decoction on the affected parts.

6) Pruritus Vulvae or Pruritus Ani

Kǔ shēn (Radix Sophorae Flavescentis), *shé chuáng zǐ* (Fructus Cnidii), *shí liú pí* (Pericarpium Granati) and *míng fán* (Alaum) are decocted in water, apply the decoction to wash the affected parts.

(Edited by Guang An Men Hospital of Academy Institute of Chinese Medicine. *Clinical Experience Collection of Zhu Ren-kang* 朱仁康临床经验集. People's Medical Publishing House 人民卫生出版社, 1979, 10)

2. Zhang Zhi-li's Combined Method of Differentiation of both Disease and Syndrome

Pruritus is hard to cure because of its complicated etiological factors. Therefore, Zhang Zhi-li emphasizes that when diagnosing and treating pruritus, find the etiological factors. Then cure combine methods of differentiating both the disease and syndrome.

1) Pruritus senilis is often caused by blood deficiency and wind dryness failing to nourish the skin. Qi and blood are interdependent. Qi deficiency causes blood obstruction and then blood deficiency fails to nourish the skin. Pruritus happens in spring and winter. It manifests as dry skin, thickening and itching.

The treatment principle is to tonify blood and moisten the skin and expel wind to relieve itching. Commonly used Chinese herbs are: *Dǎng shēn* (Radix Codonopsis), *huáng qí* (Radix Astragali), *shēng dì huáng* (Radix Rehmanniae Recens), *shú dì huáng* (Radix Rehmanniae Praeparata), *tiān mén dōng* (Radix Asparagi), *mài mén dōng* (Radix Ophiopogonis), *dāng guī* (Radix Angelicae Sinensis), *chì sháo* (Radix Paeoniae Rubra), *bái sháo* (Radix Paeoniae Alba), *yè jiāo téng* (Caulis Polygoni Multiflori), *dān shēn* (Radix et Rhizoma Salviae Miltiorrhizae), *jī xuè téng* (Caulis Spatholobi), *fáng fēng* (Radix Saposhnikoviae), *cì jí lí* (Fructus Trbuli), *kǔ shēn* (Radix Sophorae Flavescentis), *dì fū zǐ* (Fructus Kochiae) and *fú píng* (Herba Spirodelae). For winter pruritus in older people, *fú píng* (Herba Spirodelae) has unique actions of diaphoresis and dispersing exterior pathogens, expelling wind to relieve itching, and also functions to harmonize the defensive qi and nutrient qi.

In addition, the internal factors of pruritus senilis (pruritus in old age) are usually related to diseases such as neurasthenia, arteriosclerosis, diabetes, uremia and tumors. For this reason, clinical examinations should be detailed to differentiate the earliest stages of the primary pathology in accordance with the symptoms.

2) Pruritus that happens in the summer and autumn among young people is frequently caused by retention of wind-damp and malnutrition of the skin. Symptoms of the disease are whole body itching and thickening of the skin. The symptoms are also lingering and protracted. Patients of this kind usually fall ill because of improper diet and exposure to wind after drinking. Therefore smoking, wine, strong tea, spicy and fishy food are probable significant internal causative factors. The principles of treatment are expelling wind and removing dampness, tonifying blood and moistening skin.

Chinese medicinals such as *quán xiē* (Scorpio), *zào jiǎo cì* (Spina Gleditsiae), *cì jí lí* (Fructus Trbuli), *kǔ shēn* (Radix Sophorae Flavescentis), *bái xiān pí* (Cortex Dictamni), *chē qián zǐ* (Semen Plantaginis), *zé xiè* (Rhizoma Alismatis), *dì fū zǐ* (Fructus Kochiae), *bái zhú* (Rhizoma Atractylodis Macrocephalae), *zhǐ qiào* (Fructus Aurantii), *shēng dì huáng* (Radix Rehmanniae Recens), *huái huā* (Flos Sophorae), *dāng guī* (Radix Angelicae Sinensis), *yè jiāo téng* (Caulis Polygoni Multiflori), *jī xuè téng* (Caulis Spatholobi), *dān shēn* (Radix et Rhizoma Salviae Miltiorrhizae), *chì sháo* (Radix Paeoniae Rubra) and *chán tuì* (Periostracum Cicadae) are commonly used.

Pruritus vulvae is related to diseases such as profuse leucorrhea, trichomonas vaginalis, vaginal fungus diseases and uterine cervical cancer. Because of the different syndromes, a careful differentiation must be made. For syndromes of dampness due to Spleen deficiency use *shēng bái zhú* (raw Rhizoma Atractylodis Macrocephalae), *shēng zhǐ qiào* (raw Fructus Aurantii), *shēng yì yǐ rén* (raw Semen Coicis), *bì xiè* (Rhizoma Yam), *lóng dǎn cǎo* (Radix Gentianae), *shēng dì huáng* (Radix Rehmanniae Recens), *huáng bǎi* (Cortex Phellodendri), *fáng fēng* (Radix Saposhnikoviae), *kǔ shēn* (Radix Sophorae Flavescentis), *bái xiān pí* (Cortex Dictamni), *chē qián zǐ* (Semen Plantaginis), *chē qián cǎo* (Herba Plantaginis), *zé xiè* (Rhizoma Alismatis), *dāng guī* (Radix Angelicae Sinensis), *yè jiāo téng* (Caulis Polygoni Multiflori). The syndrome of parasites caused by the accumulation of damp-heat in the body and pruritus ani are both related to precipitating factors such as pinworm. Therefore a careful examination must be made in order to find the appropriate treatment for killing the parasites.

3) Apply external therapy corresponding to the differentiation of syndromes and signs. For retention of internal damp-heat, secondary infections after scratching and red and swollen of damaged skin, *Mǎ Chǐ Xiàn Xǐ Jì* (马齿苋洗剂) is used. For severe itching, decoct *chǔ shí zǐ* (Fructus Broussonetiae), *shé chuáng zǐ* (Fructus Cnidii), *cè bǎi yè* (Cacumen Platycladi), *kǔ shēn* (Radix Sophorae Flavescentis) and *dì fū zǐ* (Fructus

Kochiae) in water for external wash. For pruritus ani and external genitalia, use *Shé Chuáng Zǐ Xǐ Jì* (蛇床子洗剂) for sitz bath (demibain), which consists of *wēi líng xiān* (Radix et Rhizoma Clematidis) 15g, *shé chuáng zǐ* (Fructus Cnidii) 15g, *dāng guī wěi* (Radix Angelicae Sinensis End) 15g, *tǔ dà huáng* (Radix Rumicis Nepalensis) 15g, *kǔ shēn* (Radix Sophorae Flavescentis) 15g, *shā rén* (Fructus Amomi) and six onion bulbs.

(Edited by An Jia-feng and Zhang Bo. *Selected Zhang Zhi-li Medical Cases of Dermatogic Disease* 张志礼皮肤病医案选萃. People 's Medical Publishing House 人民卫生出版社, 1994: 158)

3. Xu Yi-hou's Combined and Simultaneous Treatment of Enriching Yin and Dispersing the Exterior

Comprehension for the History of Various Diseases (杂病源流犀烛, *Zá Bìng Yuán Liú Xī Zhú*):

血虚之痒，虫行皮中；皮虚之痒，淫淫不已；风邪之痒，痒甚难忍；酒后之痒，痒如风疮，常搔至血出。

"Itching caused by blood deficiency is just like worms crawling between the muscles and skin; itching caused by deficiency of fur skin and by pathogenic wind is hard to bear; and itching due to drinking is like itching of wind herpes, and often leads to scratch until bleeding."

Although Shen's words cannot conclude whole symptoms of itching, he had a pertinent differentiation of pruritus, therefore, it can be regarded as main points of differentiation of general pruritus.

Generally speaking, local pruritus mainly calls for external treatment, while general pruritus attaches importance to internal treatment. There are close relations between itching and wind pathogens. But using too many herbs for dispersing wind is to be avoided. This is because wind herbs are likely to consume yin and blood and thus unable to nourish the skin. Not only will the itching not be relieved, but can continue and intensify greatly.

The origin of pruritus is deficiency, wind, heat and damp. The principle of treatment is the simultaneous treatment of enriching yin and dispersing the exterior. The formula is *Shǒu Wū Qī Huā Tāng* (首乌七花汤), consisting of *hé shǒu wū* (Radix Polygoni Multiflori) 10g, *shēng dì huáng* (Radix Rehmanniae Recens) 10g, *shú dì huáng* (Radix Rehmanniae Praeparata) 10g, *gōu téng* (Ramulus Uncariae Cum Uncis) 10g, *háng jú huā* (Flos Chrysanthemi) 10g, *fáng fēng* (Radix Saposhnikoviae) 6g, *líng xiāo huā* (Flos Campsis) 6g, *huái huā* (Flos Sophorae) 6g, *hóng huā* (Flos Carthami) 6g, *méi guī huā* (Flos Rosae Rugosae) 6g, *bái biǎn dòu huā* (Flos Lablab Album) 6g, *jī guān huā* (Flos Celosiae Cristatae) 6g.

(Xu Yi-hou: Editor-in-chief. *Miracle Prescriptions of Great Physician* 名医奇方秘术 . China Medical Technology Publishing House 中国医药科技出版社 . 1995, 12)

PERSPECTIVES OF INTEGRATIVE MEDICINE

Challenges and Solutions

Challenge #1: How to Better Control the Relapse of Pruritus Senilis

Cutaneous pruritus is a common disease in dermatology, and the condition can be controlled and improved by a combined treatment of Chinese medicine and modern medicine. However, a few kinds of pruritus, such as pruritus senilis, pruritus ani and pruritus vulvae and especially pruritus resulting from internal diseases, are hard to cure, often attacking repeatedly. Itching of these kinds is difficult to control by drugs, and has become difficult issues clinically. Pruritus senilis mainly is related to hypofunction of sex hormone secretions and the sebiferous glands, asteatosis cutis, analosis and degeneration. Though medication can improve symptoms of pruritus senilis temporarily, patients will return to the former condition after withdrawal of the drug, and can be worse in autumn and winter.

To improve pruritus senilis, first of all, identify and then avoid common causes such as excessive bathing, overheated water or too many detergent. These are all common causes of the disease. Instruct patients that after washing to use moisturizers, such as *shā shēn* (Radix Glehniae), *yù zhú* (Rhizoma Polygonati Odorati), *yín ěr* (Tremella Fuciformis) and "snow frogs". Eat some fatty meat if possible. If itching is serious, consider estrogen hormone treatment. Be vigilant to exclude internal diseases, especially hidden issues like tumors.

Challenge #2: Treating Pruritus Ani and External Genitalia

In the clinic, pruritus of the external genitalia is most commonly seen among middle-aged people. A considerable amount of patients get treatment but without obvious improvement, or else they quickly relapse. They become obsessed and self-diagnosis themselves that they have acquired a venereal disease and frequently do venereal examinations. They may frequently soak the affected parts in external washes and thus aggravate the condition. This results in more anxiety, insomnia and emotion changes. Sufferers of this kind tend to be women patients. Under this condition, detailed examinations first must be made to exclude candida (monilia) and ciliaphora protozoas (infusorian). Instruct the patient not to use irritating agents, such as detergents and (inappropriate) topical medicated solutions. After every defecation, clean the genital area with clean water. Patients should not wear synthetic underwear pants and they should be kept cool and loose.

Besides conventional treatment, one can select acupuncture points such as DU 1 or RN 1 (*huì yīn*). For patients with emotional issues, apply sedatives and anti-anxiety medicine, such as Fluoxetine and Seroxat. Chinese medicinals for dispersing depressed Liver-qi and regulating the flow of qi, enriching Heart and calming the spirit can be used.

Challenge #3: Handling of Stubborn Pruritus

Clinically, some patients with extensive and stubborn pruritus have already taken a lot of herbs and medicine, but without improvement. For this kind of patient a detailed medical examination must be made. During the early stage of primary biliary cirrhosis, extensive pruritus may appear. Cholestyramine is helpful to treat pruritus of cholestasia. Chronic renal failure may lead to pruritus, obvious during or after dialysis and the causative factors of toxuria patients include asteatosis cutis, Mastocytosis and increasing blood magnesium.

Pruritus seen with cancer is relatively rare. (However in Hodgkin's disease it can approach 30%.) It is, however, an important sign that may be seen long before other clinical symptoms of disease. Extremely severe pruritus indicates an unfavorable prognosis and accelerating pathogenetic conditions. For obstinate pruritus due to internal diseases, active treatment of primary etiological factors will improve itching symptoms effectively. One should also be aware that some stubborn pruritus occurs because of neurosis or anxiety. For this reason, psychological treatment should be used concurrently.

Challenge #4: How to Achieve Integrative Medicine

Practitioners of Chinese medicine think of pruritus as being caused by the invasion of exopathogenic wind-cold or wind-heat. It can be a functional disorder of the viscera (*zang* and *fu* organs) from blood-heat or damp-heat encumbering. It may also be a Liver and Kidney deficiency due to old age and the resulting blood deficiency and wind dryness. Doctors of biomedicine understand that there are complications of both external and internal etiological factors. Integrative medicine will do patients a lot of good in improving their quality of life.

When a patient's condition is serious, antihistamine drugs should be used to control it. At the same time, the pattern differentiation of the syndrome should be the foundation of combining traditional Chinese medicinals. This can shorten the antihistamine treatment time, relieve side effects due to their long-term use, and reduce the chances of relapse. When treating the disease by Chinese medicinals, modern medical methods such as isotopes, ultraviolet and superficial X-ray therapy can also be applied. Excellent results can be expected in treating pruritus with integrative medicine.

Insight from Empirical Wisdom

1. Doctors should examine the causes of pruritus in detail, and look into etiological factors as well as excluding local ones.

Take this case for example: A patient with pruritus vulvae had for years taken many prescriptions and applied hormone ointments for external use, but had stopped improving. At first, the doctor did not notice it, but after careful examination, he detected crab louses in the pubic hair and some were active. With symptomatic treatment, the patient recovered in a week.

Another patient with hemorrhoids had obstinate and lingering perianal itching. After curing the hemorrhoid, the perianal itch was cured spontaneously. For example, pruritus in winter is often aggravated by excessive bathing with too hot water and can be improved only through correcting the causative factors. All of these can not take effect unless doctors find the etiological factors and carefully treat with a differentiation of the syndromes.

2. Doctors should take the time and initiative to help patients with instructions and to guide patients psychologically if necessary. Many kinds of pruritus have a connection with an external environmental factor. So it calls upon doctors to instruct patients to refrain from them, to eat properly and to participate in their own treatment. These play an

important role in treatment. Some patients suffer from long-term itching, thus causing even more anxiety. The more they scratch, the more itching they feel. For these patients with emotional issues, doctors should give psychological guidance and persuade them not to scratch.

3. Prescribing medicine by the differentiation of syndromes, gives simultaneous treatment of both the symptoms and the root. Although all the patients have itching there may be different reasons for it. If the physician blindly goes after only stopping the itching it may not necessarily be effective. This is especially true when applying Chinese medicinals. For older people, the syndromes are usually yin deficiency, blood deficiency and blood dryness, so the principle is primarily enriching blood and moistening dryness.

Chinese medicinals such as *jī xuè téng* (Caulis Spatholobi), *hé shǒu wū* (Radix Polygoni Multiflori), *shú dì huáng* (Radix Rehmanniae Praeparata), *mài mén dōng* (Raidix Ophiopogonis), *yù zhú* (Rhizoma Polygonati Odorati) and *wǔ wèi zǐ* (Fructus Schisandrae), or *nǚ zhēn zǐ* (Fructus Ligustri Lucidi), *hàn lián cǎo* (Herba Ecliptae), *shēng dì huáng* (Radix Rehmanniae Recens), *tài zǐ shēn* (Radix Pseudostellariae), *zhī mǔ* (Rhizoma Anemarrhenae) are used for enriching yin and moistening dryness, then assisted by dispelling wind and relieving itching. Pay special attention not to dispel dampness arbitrarily, for the impairment of yin causes dryness and skin itching. There are eliminating-wind medicinals for treating pruritus, but dispersing too much will consume the yin fluids. For obstinate and prolonged pruritus, add *wū shāo shé* (Zaocys), *quán xiē* (Scorpio), *wú gōng* (Scolopendra) for removing wind and communicating collaterals, removing wind to relieve itching.

Summary

Cutaneous pruritus is a common and multiple faceted dermatogic disease characterized by skin itching. Because of a lack of a convenient technology for measuring itching, there is little research on the molecular basis, pathologic physiology and therapy, so no ideal therapy for relieving itching can be chosen at this time. Pruritus is caused by many factors, removal of irritating factors being an important part during treatment. Due to the complicated etiological factors of some pruritus, seeking or eliminating of them is difficult.

The existing therapy adopted by biomedicine is applying anti-inflammatory agents, such as corticosteroid and antihistamine drugs. However, the action of resisting itching is accompanied by anti-inflammatory actions, and is unable to cure pruritus completely. Furthermore, long-term use of cortical hormone can bring side effects. Traditional H1 receptor antagonist has obvious effect of sedation, affecting its applying range. New H1 receptor antagonist without sedation has not been applied extensively yet.

The course of treatment of Chinese medicine is comparatively long, but has a long-term alleviating therapeutic effect for gentle and medium pruritus. For severe pruritus, especially caused by internal diseases, applying integrative medicine will achieve fine results. The major subject at present is how to improve itching symptoms quickly and lasting. We should further look for and choose prescriptions with exact therapeutic effect, and continue to research etiology and etiopathogenesis. And it is urgent for us to explore the nature of pruritus with integrative treatment.

Chinese medicine has its advantages in treating and regulating cutaneous pruritus and making effective treatment according to patients' constitution and symptoms. For young people falling ill in summer, the principle is mainly to clear heat and dispel dampness, expel wind and relieve itching. For old and middle-aged people, one should put emphasis on regulating and enriching qi and blood, dispelling wind and relieving itching.

Clinical manifestations of pruritus are relatively simple, so it is easy to diagnose. The key point is to look for and then exclude etiological factors. Both doctors of Chinese medicine and biomedicine consider that there are multiple etiological factors of pruritus. They are general or local, caused by exterior or interior factors, or with no internal factors. For this reason, to treat pruritus, doctors must first search for the etiological factors. The basic principle of treating pruritus is to identify the different etiology of the disease, (and treating correspondingly) while considering both the root causes and symptoms.

SELECTED QUOTES FROM CLASSICAL TEXTS

Basic Questions - True and Great Comments (素问 · 至真要大论 , *Sù Wèn·Zhì Zhēn Yào Dà Lùn*):

诸痛痒疮，皆属于心。

"All pains and pruritus originate form Heart."

Treatise on the Causes and Manifestations of Diseases - Manifestations of Wind Itch (诸病源候论 · 风瘙痒候 , *Zhū Bìng Yuán Hòu Lùn·Fēng Sāo Yǎng Hòu*):

风瘙痒者，是体虚受风，风入腠理，与血气相搏，而俱往来于皮肤之间。邪气微，不能冲击为痛，故但瘙痒也。

"Cutaneous pruritus is caused by wind invasion of weak body into the striae and interstitial space, fighting with qi and blood, and then alternating between interstices of the skin. Minor pathogens will not impact as pain, so it manifests as itching."

Treatise on the Causes and Manifestations of Diseases - Manifestations of Wind Itch (诸病源候论 · 风瘙痒候 , *Zhū Bìng Yuán Hòu Lùn·Gǔ Dào Yǎng Hòu*):

谷道痒者，由胃弱肠虚，则蛲虫下侵谷道，重者食于肛门，轻者但痒也，蛲虫状极细微，形如今之虫状也。

"Anal itching is caused by weak stomach and intestine, pinworm attacking downward into anus, biting anus if ill severely, only causing itching if slightly ill. Pinworms are extremely tiny, just like parasites nowadays."

The Golden Mirror of Medicine - Mental Cultivation Methods and Significance Trick of Surgery (医宗金鉴 · 外科心法要诀 , *Yī Zōng Jīn Jiàn·Wài Kē Xīn Fǎ Yào Jué*):

小儿肛门作痒，由虫蚀也。

"Childhood pruritus ani is caused by biting worms."

Whole Book for Syndrome Differentiation and Treatment of Surgery - Wind-itch (外科证治全书 · 痒风 , *Wài Kē Zhèng Zhì Quán Shū·Yǎng Fēng*):

遍身瘙痒，并无疮疥，瘙之不止。

"For itching all over the body without sores and scabies, one can not help scratching."

Great Achievement of Surgery - All Pruritus (外科大成 · 诸痒 , *Wài Kē Dà Chéng·Zhū Yǎng*):

诸疮痛痒，皆属于火；风盛则痒，盖为风者，火之标也，凡风热客于皮肤，作痒起粟者，治宜疏风，如换肌丸、苦参丸等；若风热内淫，血虚作痒，又当凉润燥，如逍遥散、柴胡汤之类也。

"All pains and pruritus originate from fire; hyperactivity of wind causes itching because wind is the symbol of fire, when wind-heat guesting superficial, itching with millets, treated by the principle of dispersing wind, such as *Huàn Jī Wán* (换 肌 丸) and *Kǔ Shēn Wán* (苦参丸). If wind-heat invasion is internal, itching due to blood deficiency, principle is cooling heat and moistening dryness, such as *Xiāo Yáo Sǎn* and *Chái Hú Tāng* (柴胡汤)."

Whole Book for Syndrome Differentiation and Treatment of Surgery · Wind-Itch (外科证治全书 · 痒风 , *Wài Kē Zhèng Zhì Quán Shū·Yǎng Fēng*):

肝家血虚，燥热生风，不可妄投风药。

"Patients suffering from liver disease have deficiency in blood, dryness and heat generating wind, for this kind of patients, use wind medicinals cautiously."

MODERN RESEARCH

Clinical Research

1. Pattern Differentiation and Corresponding Treatment

(1) Chen classified cutaneous pruritus into two categories, patterns of excess and deficiency. Excess patterns include patterns of wind hyperactivity, wind-cold, wind-heat, wind-damp, blood heat, damp-heat, damp invasion of lower *Jiao* and blood stasis.

For wind hyperactivity pattern, the principle is relieving muscles and dispersing exterior, expelling wind and relieving itching, formula is *Wū Shé Qū Fēng Tāng* (乌蛇驱风汤).

For wind-cold pattern, principle is dispelling wind and removing cold, balancing *ying* and *wei* qi, formula is modified *Guì Zhī Má Huáng Gè Bàn Tāng* (桂枝麻黄各半汤).

For wind-heat types, the principle is clearing heat and resolve toxinsing to dispel wind and relieve itching. The formula is *Xiāo Fēng Sǎn* (消风散).

For wind-damp patterns, the principle is expelling wind and eliminating dampness, coordinating ying and relieving itching. The formula is *Qiāng Huó Shèng Shī Tāng* (羌活胜湿汤).

For blood heat types, the principle is clearing heat and cooling blood, dispersing wind and relieving itching. The formula is modified *Dì Sháo Liáng Xuè Tāng* (地芍凉血汤).

For damp-heat types, the principle is clearing heat and drying dampness, milding middle and relieving itching. The formula is modified *Bì Xiè Shèn Shī Tāng* (革薢渗湿汤).

For a damp invasion of the lower *jiao*, the principle is clearing heat and purging Liver, eliminating dampness to relieve itching. The formula is modified *Lóng Dăn Xiè Gān Tāng* (龙胆泻肝汤).

For blood stasis types, the principle is invigorating blood and transforming stasis, eliminating wind to relieve itching and the formula is *Táo Hóng Sì Wù Tāng* (桃红四物汤).

Deficiency patterns include blood deficiency, Liver and Kidney yin deficiency.

For blood deficiency, the principle is enriching blood and moistening dryness, extinguishing wind to relieve itching. The formula is *Sì Wù Xiāo Fēng Tāng* (四物消风汤) or *Shū Fēng Yăng Xuè Tāng* (疏风养血汤).

For pattern of Liver and Kidney yin deficiency, the principle is tonifying Liver and Kidney, extinguishing wind to relieve itching. The formulas are *Zhī Băi Dì Huáng Wán* (知柏地黄丸) or modified *Gān Shèn Liăng Zī Tāng* (肝肾两滋汤). [1]

(2) Wang classified pruritus into 5 categories:

For a blood heat pattern, use *Yăng Xuè Qū Fēng Tāng* (养血祛风汤).

For a blood stasis pattern, use *Huó Xuè Qū Fēng Tāng* (活血祛风汤).

For a wind and damp-heat invasion pattern, use *Wū Shé Qū Fēng Tāng*.

For an invasion of external wind-cold, use *Guì Zhī Má Huáng Tāng* (桂枝麻黄汤).

For yin deficiency of Liver and Kidney use *Yăng Xuè Xī Fēng Tāng* (养血熄风汤). [2]

(3) Han classified pruritus into 2 categories:

For wind-heat and blood-heat, the principle is expelling wind and clearing heat, assisted by cooling blood to relieve itching. The formula is modified *Sì Wù Tāng* (四物汤).

For blood deficiency and Liver hyperactivity, the principle is enriching blood and expelling wind, moistening dryness to relieve itching. The formula is modified *Dāng Guī Yǐn Zi* (当归饮子). Treating 60 cases, the total effective rate was 92.5%. [3]

2. Specific Formulas

(1) Prescription for Internal Treatment

1) *Yǎng Xuè Rùn Fū Tāng* (养血润肤汤)

Dān shēn (Radix et Rhizoma Salviae Miltiorrhizae) 15g, *chì sháo* (Radix Paeoniae Rubra) 15g, *bái sháo* (Raidix Paeoniae Alba) 15g, *shēng dì huáng* (Radix Rehmanniae) 15g, *shú dì huáng* (Radix Rehmanniae Praeparata) 15g, *bǎi zǐ rén* (Semen Platycladi) 15g, *shí chāng pú* (Rhizoma Acori Tatarinowii) 15g, *chuān xiōng* (Rhizoma Chuanxiong) 10g, *wū shāo shé* (Zaocys) 10g, *hóng huā* (Flos Carthami) 3g, *yè jiāo téng* (Caulis Polygoni Multiflori) 30g, *cì jí lí* (Fructus Trbuli) 30g, *quán guā lóu* (Fructus Trichosanthis) 30g.

For constipation, add *shú dì huáng* (Radix Rehmanniae Praeparata) 10g.

For irritable patients with chest and hypochondrium pain and flatulence, add *lóng dǎn cǎo* (Radix Gentianae) 10g and *chái hú* (Radix Bupleuri) 10g.

For poor quality of sleeping, add *chǎo zǎo rén* (Semen Ziziphi Spinosae Tosum) 10g and *hé huān pí* (Cortex Albiziae) 15g.

For poor appetite, add *bái zhú* (Rhizoma Atractylodis Macrocephalae) 10g and *huái shān yào* (Rhizoma Dioscoreae) 30g.

For protracted disease, add *quán xiē* (Scorpio) 6g, *zào jiǎo cì* (Spina Gleditsiae). In treating 60 cases of pruritus senilis, the total effective rate reached 95.0%. [4]

2) *Jiǔ Xiān Tāng* (韭仙汤)

Jiǔ zǐ (Semen Allii Tuberosi) 10g, *yín yáng huò* (Herba Epimedii) 10g, *shí nán yè* (Folium Photiniae) 10g, *gān cǎo* (Radix and Rhizoma Glycyrrhizae)

8g. In treating 63 cases of pruritus senilis simplex, the total effective rate reached 92.1%. [5]

3) *Rùn Fū Zhǐ Yǎng Tāng* (润肤止痒汤)

Dāng guī (Radix Angelicae Sinensis) 10g, *hé shǒu wū* (Radix Polygoni Multiflori) 10g, *fáng fēng* (Radix Saposhnikoviae) 10g, *qín jiāo* (Radix Gentianae Macrophyllae) 10g, *huáng qí* (Radix Astragali) 20g, *cì jí lí* (Fructus Trbuli) 30g, *bái xiān pí* (Cortex Dictamni) 30g, *jīng jiè* (Herba Schizonepetae) 10g, *bái sháo* (Raidix Paeoniae Alba) 10g, *chuān xiōng* (Rhizoma Chuanxiong) 10g, *shú dì huáng* (Radix Rehmanniae Praeparata) 10g, *gān cǎo* (Radix et Rhizoma Glycyrrhizae) 10g. In treating 35 cases of pruritus senilis, the total effective rate reached 77.15%. [6]

4) *QuánXiē Zhǐ Yǎng Tāng* (全蝎止痒汤)

Quán xiē (Scorpio) 9g, *zào jiǎo cì* (Spina Gleditsiae) 9g, *shé chuáng zǐ* (Fructus Cnidii) 15g, *shēng dì huáng* (Radix Rehmanniae Recens) 30g, *shú dì huáng* (Radix Rehmanniae Praeparata) 30g, *fáng fēng* (Radix Saposhnikoviae) 30g, *dāng guī* (Radix Angelicae Sinensis) 20g, *dān shēn* (Radix et Rhizoma Salviae Miltiorrhizae) 20g, *hé shǒu wū* (Radix Polygoni Multiflori) 20g, *bái xiān pí* (Cortex Dictamni) 20g, *cì jí lí* (Fructus Trbuli) 20g. Decoct all the above medicinals in water 2 times, the first decoction for oral use, the second decoction for external use. Treating 37 cases of pruritus senilis, satisfactory results had been achieved. [7]

5) Modified *Guì Zhī Tāng* (桂枝汤)

Guì zhī (Ramulus Cinnamomi) 15g, *chǎo bái sháo* (Raidix Paeoniae Alba Tosum) 15g, *hé shǒu wū* (Radix Polygoni Multiflori) 15g, *fáng fēng* (Radix Saposhnikoviae) 15g, *shēng jiāng* (Rhizoma Zingiberis Recens) 6g, *dà zǎo* (Fructus Jujubae) 6 pieces, *gān cǎo* (Radix et Rhizoma Glycyrrhizae) 7g. In treating 58 cases of pruritus senilis, the total effective rate reached 93.0%. [8]

6) *Yǎng Xuè Rùn Fū Yǐn* (养血润肤饮)

Dǎng shēn (Radix Codonopsis) 10g, *huáng qí* (Radix Astragali) 10g, *shēng dì huáng* (Radix Rehmanniae Recens) 10g, *shú dì huáng* (Radix Rehmanniae Praeparata) 10g, *mài mén dōng* (Raidix Ophiopogonis) 10g, *dāng guī* (Radix Angelicae Sinensis) 10g, *chì sháo* (Radix Paeoniae Rubra) 10g, *bái sháo* (Raidix Paeoniae Alba) 10g, *dān shēn* (Radix et Rhizoma Salviae Miltiorrhizae) 15g, *jī xuè téng* (Caulis Spatholobi) 15g, *yè jiāo téng* (Caulis Polygoni Multiflori) 30g, *fáng fēng* (Radix Saposhnikoviae) 10g, *cì jí lí* (Fructus Trbuli) 30g, *kǔ shēn* (Radix Sophorae Flavescentis) 15g, *dì fū zǐ* (Fructus Kochiae) 15g, and *fú píng* (Herba Spirodelae) 10g. [9]

7) *Huáng qí* (Radix Astragali) 30g, *dǎng shēn* (Radix Codonopsis) 15g, *dāng guī* (Radix Angelicae Sinensis) 20g, *bái zhú* (Rhizoma Atractylodis Macrocephalae) 15g, *cāng zhú* (Rhizoma Atractylodis) 15g, *chì sháo* (Radix Paeoniae Rubra) 15g, *bái sháo* (Raidix Paeoniae Alba) 15g, *fáng fēng* (Radix Saposhnikoviae) 10g, *huáng bǎi* (Cortex Phellodendri) 10g, *shēng má* (Rhizoma Cimicifugae) 3g, *chái hú* (Radix Bupleuri) 10g, *chén pí* (Pericarpium Citri Reticulatae) 10g. Decoct the herbs in water twice, for both oral and external use, 1 packet per day.

Kǔ shēn (Radix Sophorae Flavescentis) 20g, *fáng fēng* (Radix Saposhnikoviae) 15g, *dì fū zǐ* (Fructus Kochiae) 15g, *huáng bǎi* (Cortex Phellodendri) 10g, *bǎi bù* (Radix Stemonae) 10g, decoct above herbs in water for washing, 2 times , 1 packet per day. In treating 20 cases of stubborn pruritus ani, 12 cases were cured and 6 cases improved. [10]

8) *Bǔ Xīn Tāng* (补心汤)

Shēng dì huáng (Radix Rehmanniae Recens) 12g, *wǔ wèi zǐ* (Fructus Schisandrae) 10g, *dāng guī* (Radix Angelicae Sinensis) 12g, *tiān dōng* (Radix Asparagi) 10g, *mài mén dōng* (Raidix Ophiopogonis) 10g, *suān zǎo rén* (Semen Ziziphi Spinosae) 10g, *dǎng shēn* (Radix Codonopsis) 12g, *xuán shēn* (Raidix Scrophulariae) 10g, *dān shēn* (Radix et Rhizoma

Salviae Miltiorrhizae) 15g, *fú líng* (Poria) 12g, *gān cǎo* (Radix and Rhizoma Glycyrrhizae) 9g.

For complications by a simultaneous invasion of external wind, add *fáng fēng* (Radix Saposhnikoviae) 6g, *dì fū zǐ* (Fructus Kochiae) 9g. For yin deficiency and dry intestines, add *zhì shǒu wū* (Prepared Radix Polygoni Multiflori) 9g, *hú má rén* (Semen Cannabis) 9g.

For heat in the blood phase, add *bái sháo* (Raidix Paeoniae Alba) 12g, *mǔ dān pí* (Cortex Moutan) 12g. In treating 72 cases of pruritus senilis vulvae, the total effective rate reached 97.2%. [11]

9) *Yǎng Xuè Róu Gān Huà Yū Tāng* (养血柔肝化瘀汤)

Shēng dì huáng (Radix Rehmanniae Recens) 15g, *zhì shǒu wū* (Radix Polygoni Multiflori Praeparata) 15g, *chì sháo* (Radix Paeoniae Rubra) 15g, *dān pí* (Cortex Moutan) 15g, *cì jí lí* (Fructus Trbuli) 15g, *dān shēn* (Radix et Rhizoma Salviae Miltiorrhizae) 20g, *yè jiāo téng* (Caulis Polygoni Multiflori) 20g, *suān zǎo rén* (Semen Ziziphi Spinosae) 20g, *jī xuè téng* (Caulis Spatholobi) 20g, *táo rén* (Semen Persicae) 6g, *hóng huā* (Flos Carthami) 6g, *quán xiē* (Scorpio) 6g, *chǎo bái sháo* (Stirred Raidix Paeoniae Alba) 10g, *fú líng* (Poria) 10g, *zhēn zhū mǔ* (Concha Margaritifera) 30g, *gān cǎo* (Radix and Rhizoma Glycyrrhizae) 6g. In treating 62 cases of pruritus senilis, the total effective rate reached 90.32%. [12]

10) Modified *Dāng Guī Yǐn Zi* (当归饮子)

In treating 78 and 36 cases of pruritus senilis vulvae, the total effective rate was 96.15% and 97% separately. [13][14]

11) Additional Formulas Research

a. Zhang Guo-an, under the guide-line of "treating blood prior to treating wind", created *Xuè Fēng Tāng* (血风汤), consisting of *shēng dì huáng* (Radix Rehmanniae Recens), *mǔ dān pí* (Cortex Moutan), *chì sháo* (Radix Paeoniae Rubra), *bái sháo* (Raidix Paeoniae Alba), *hé shǒu wū*

(Radix Polygoni Multiflori), *zǐ cǎo* (Radix Arnebiae), *chán tuì* (Periostracum Cicadae), *bái jí lí* (Fructus Trbuli), *dān shēn* (Radix et Rhizoma Salviae Miltiorrhizae), *gān cǎo* (Radix and Rhizoma Glycyrrhizae), in treating 52 cases, proved entirely effective. [15]

b. Yang Xue-jing applied *Rùn Fū Zhǐ Yǎng Tāng*（润肤止痒汤）, which consisted of *shǒu wū téng* (Caulis Polygoni Multiflori), *jī xuè téng* (Caulis Spatholobi), *shēng dì huáng* (Radix Rehmanniae Recens), *shú dì huáng* (Radix Rehmanniae Praeparata), *dāng guī* (Radix Angelicae Sinensis), *chì sháo* (Radix Paeoniae Rubra), *bái sháo* (Raidix Paeoniae Alba), *fáng fēng* (Radix Saposhnikoviae), *cì jí lí* (Fructus Trbuli), *kǔ shēn* (Radix Sophorae Flavescentis), to treat pruritus senilis 30 cases, 24 cases fully recovered, 2 cases turned out to be effective, 4 cases improved. [16]

c. Liu Zong-yan prescribed *Dān Jī Yín Qiào Yǐn* (丹鸡银翘饮), which consisted of *dān shēn* (Radix et Rhizoma Salviae Miltiorrhizae), *jī xuè téng* (Caulis Spatholobi), *jīn yín huā* (Flos Lonicerae), *lián qiào* (Fructus Forsythiae), *dāng guī* (Radix Angelicae Sinensis), *chuān xiōng* (Rhizoma Chuanxiong), *chì bái sháo* (Radix Paeoniae Rubra and Alba), *shēng dì huáng* (Radix Rehmanniae Recens), *jīng jiè suì* (Spica Schizonepetae), *fáng fēng* (Radix Saposhnikoviae), *dì fū zǐ* (Fructus Kochiae), and *bò hé* (Herba Menthae). To treat 80 cases of pruritus, setting up 50 comparison groups applying 4 mg Cyproheptadine and 0.2mg vitamin C orally 3 times a day, with intravenous 10ml 10% calglucon in 20ml 50% GS. Effective rate of the treatment group was 98.19%, comparison group 60%. [17]

d. Hu Zhi-fang created *Èr Chóng Sì Wù Tāng* (二虫四物汤), which consisted of *shú dì huáng* (Radix Rehmanniae Praeparata), *yè jiāo téng* (Caulis Polygoni Multiflori), *bái sháo* (Radix Paeoniae Rubra), *dāng guī* (Radix Angelicae Sinensis), *chuān xiōng* (Rhizoma Chuanxiong), *wū shāo shé* (Zaocys), *chán tuì* (Periostracum Cicadae), *fáng fēng* (Radix Saposhnikoviae), and *cì jí lí* (Fructus Trbuli). All of the 15 cases of pruritus senilis he treated were cured. [18]

e. Yin Chuan-kai used *Dāng Guī Yǐn Zi Hé Sì Zhòng Tāng* (当归饮子合四重汤) (*cí shí* (Magnetitum), *dài zhě shí* (Ocherum Rubrum), *zhēn zhū mǔ* (Concha Margaritifera), *mǔ lì* (Concha Ostreae)) to treat 48 cases of pruritus senilis, effective rate was 91.17%.[19]

f. Xu Xiu-rong used *Biàn Tōng Guī Pí Tāng* (变通归脾汤), consisting of *dǎng shēn* (Radix Codonopsis), *huáng qí* (Radix Astragali), *quán dāng guī* (Radix Angelicae Sinensis), *fú shén* (Poria), *bái zhú* (Rhizoma Atractylodis Macrocephalae), *lóng yǎn ròu* (Arillus Longan), *suān zǎo rén* (Semen Ziziphi Spinosae), *yuǎn zhì* (Radix Polygalae), *zhì shǒu wū* (Radix Polygoni Multiflori Praeparata), *cí shí* (Magnetitum), *zhì jí lí* (Fructus Trbuli Praeparata), *fáng fēng* (Radix Saposhnikoviae), *zhì gān cǎo* (Radix et Rhizoma Glycyrrhizae Praeparata cum Melle). In treating 50 cases of pruritus senilis he set up a 50 person western medicine comparison group, applying 4mg chlorphenamine orally, Tid, 20mg Vitamine E, Bid, Vitamine C 0.2g, Tid. Effective rates were 94%, 74% respectively. [20]

(2) Formulas for External Use

1) *Míng Fán Kǔ Jiāo Xūn Xǐ Jì* (明矾苦椒熏洗剂)

Kǔ shēn (Radix Sophorae Flavescentis) 40g, *huā jiāo* (Pericarpium Zanthoxyli) 40g, *bái xiān pí* (Cortex Dictamni) 30g, *huáng bǎi* (Cortex Phellodendri) 30g, *bái jí lí* (Fructus Trbuli) 30g, *tǔ fú líng* (Rhizoma Smilacis Glabrae) 30g, *dì fū zǐ* (Fructus Kochiae) 30g, *shé chuáng zǐ* (Fructus Cnidii) 30g, *míng fán* (Alaum) 15g, *xuán míng fěn* (Natrii Sulfas Exsiccatus) 60g, one packet per day, decoct in water, wash after steaming twice. Treating 68 cases of pruritus, 53 cases had fully recovered, 15 cases had a positive effect. After taking medication for 3-5 days the conditions of itching were relieved dramatically. [21]

2) *Zhǐ Yǎng Xǐ Jì* (止痒洗剂)

Dà huáng (Radix et Rhizoma Rhei) 15g, *dà fēng zǐ* (Fructus Hydnocarpus) 15g, *shé chuáng zǐ* (Fructus Cnidii) 15g, *kǔ shēn* (Radix

Sophorae Flavescentis) 15g, *ròu cóng róng* (Herba Cistanches) 15g, *dāng guī* (Radix Angelicae Sinensis) 15g, *huáng bǎi* (Cortex Phellodendri) 12g, *cāng zhú* (Rhizoma Atractylodis) 12g, *chuān xiōng* (Rhizoma Chuanxiong) 12g, *huáng qín* (Radix Scutellariae)9g, *xuán shēn* (Raidix Scrophulariae) 30g, *bīng piàn* (Broneolum Syntheticum) 3g (decoct later). Decoct the above medicinals in water for an external wash in treating 45 cases of pruritus, among which 24 cases had been cured completely, 15 cases improved, 6 cases turned out to be ineffective. [22]

3) *Shū Fū Sǎn* (舒肤散)

Kǔ shēn (Radix Sophorae Flavescentis), *huáng bǎi* (Cortex Phellodendri), *huáng lián* (Rhizoma Coptidis), *shí liú pí* (Pericarpium Granati), *shí dà gōng láo* (Folium Jilecis), *shān liǔ jú* (Herba Umbellate Hawkweed), *dì fū zǐ* (Fructus Kochiae), *dì yú* (Radix Sanguisorbae).

This prescription was created by Song Guang-ying. Soak in boiling water and use the decoction to wash the affected parts. 174 treatment pruritus cases and a comparison group of 111 persons were set up. A solution of cresol (Lysol) and soap solution with warm water (20:5000) for washing was used, 2 times a day. In ten days, all patients treated by the *Shū Fū Sǎn* (舒肤散) fully recovered, the number of healed cases in the comparison group was 78 (70.27%). [23]

4) *Liáng Xuè Huó Xuè Zhǐ Yǎng Fāng* (凉血活血止痒方)

Hóng huā (Flos Carthami) 20g, *zǐ cǎo* (Radix Arnebiae) 20g, *zhī zǐ* (Fructus Gardeniae) 20g, *dà huáng* (Radix et Rhizoma Rhei) 20g, *bīng piàn* (Broneolum Syntheticum) 5g.

Wang Wei-ping used this formula to treat 25 cases of pruritus senilis by applying herbs on the umbilicus. This was done by using *hóng huā* (Flos Carthami), *zǐ cǎo* (Radix Arnebiae), *zhī zǐ* (Fructus Gardeniae) and *dà huáng* (Radix et Rhizoma Rhei) which were dried and ground into a powder and then *bīng piàn* (Broneolum Syntheticum) was added. These were mixed with vaseline to form a paste and then made into "cakes" about 3cm×3cm×1cm. This was put on the umbilicus and then covered with a dressing. The dressing was changed once a day for no more than 15 days until recovery. The total effective rate was 96%. [24]

3. Acupuncture and Moxibustion

(1) Employing a reinforcing method by twirling the needle, Li used GV 4; DU 4 (*mìng mén*) together with bleeding of the veins of the back of the ear, the *Du* channel on top of the head and *Jing*-well and *xing*-spring points along the twelve-meridians. In treating 38 cases of pruritus, the total effective rate was 94.7%. [25]

(2) Yang used acupuncture on two categories of patients:

For a blood deficiency-Liver hyperactivity pattern use SP 10, LI 11, SP 6, LI 4 and BL 40.

For a damp-heat pattern, use ST 36, BL 57, SP 10, LI 11 and SP 9. Needle by reinforcing after reducing, once per day, ten times as a course. It was paired with bleeding of the veins at the back of the ear, and moxibustion at SP 10 and LI 11. In treating 52 cases of pruritus senilis, the effective rate was 90.38%. [26]

(3) For pruritus senilis, Tang needled SP 10, SP 6, ST 36 and ST 21. Use moxibustion on RN 8. In treating 40 cases, all had good results. [27]

(4) He Deng selected for using plum blossom *shu*-acupoints, taiyang back-shu point positive reaction areas. (First palpating the spinal column bilaterally, if there were any ropy areas or nodes or sensations of aching or numbness, it was regarded as a positive reaction.) A Chinese medicinal decoction was used for both oral use and external wash. The formula was *hé shŏu wū* (Radix Polygoni Multiflori) 20g, *shēng dì huáng* (Radix Rehmanniae) 20g, *shú dì huáng* (Radix Rehmanniae Praeparata) 20g, *bái sháo* (Raidix Paeoniae Alba) 15g, *cì jí lí* (Fructus Trbuli) 10g, *fáng fēng* (Radix Saposhnikoviae) 10g, *shé chuáng zĭ* (Fructus Cnidii) 10g, *bái*

jiāng cán (Bombyx Batryticatus) 10g, *dāng guī* (Radix Angelicae Sinensis) 10g. Decoct in water, using the first filtration for oral use, the second for washing. In treating pruritus senilis 65 cases, the total effective rate was 100%. [28]

(5) Xu used moderately warm stick moxibustion on perineal affected areas to treat pruritus ani. In 72 cases, the total effective rate was 83%. [29]

(6) Liu used implanted ear needles to treat pruritus vulvae.

For cold dampness stagnation: external genitals, urethra, anus, intertragal notch, along with shenmen, heart, small intestine.

For qi stagnation and blood stasis: external genitals, urethra, anus, along with spleen and liver.

For qi and blood deficiency: external genitals, kidney, liver, along with end of feet, shenmen.

Observing 44 cases, the effective rate was 97.7%. [30]

(7) Liu used primarily ear acupuncture therapy to treat pruritus vulvae.

For damp invasion of the lower *Jiao*: ear points of shenmen, Sanjiao, and liver, along with the body point LV3.

For insect and bacterial infection: shenmen, spleen, bladder, along with body point *Bai Chong Wo* (bilateral).

For yin deficiency and blood dryness, use stomach, uterus, endocrine, along with the body point SP 10.

Treating 80 cases, the effectiveness was 90%. [31]

(8) Zhang Jie used a protocol of taping press ear seeds to treat 63 cases of pruritus who were divided into 2 groups. Group one received: shenmen, lung, liver, endocrine. Group two received: heart, gallbladder, wind stream, adrenal gland, subcortex. Alternating the points, after taping on *wáng bù liú xíng* (Semen Vaccariae), the patients were instructed to press the points 50 times, to the extent of feeling pain, redness and warmth in the ears, 2-3 times per day. The treatment days and course

depended on different seasons. After treating for 1-2 courses of therapy, the cure rate was 93.7%, and the efficacious rate was 100%. [32]

(9) To treat pruritus Zhang Yan-li acupunctured DU 14 (*dà zhuī*), BL 15 (*xīn shù*), BL 18 (*gān shù*), BL 13 (*fèi shù*) and BL 20 (*pí shù*), etc, then cupped on the points for 10-15min, so as to extract some blood or fluid, once a day. In treating 24 cases of pruritus, 19 cases were healed completely and all were efficacious to some degree. [33]

(10) Liu Xin-jian did tapping stimulation with medium strength bilaterally on each side of the spine from the neck to the sacrum and then focused the tapping on DU 14, BL 13, BL 20, BL 21 (*wèi shù*), to make it bleed slightly. Cupping was applied to the bleeding parts for about 10-15min. Every other day, successively 3 times was considered a course. In treating 36 cases of pruritus, after 2-6 times, they were healed entirely. [34]

Experimental Studies

Research on the Efficacy of Herbal Prescriptions

(1) Clinical and Experimental Studies of *Xiān Fāng Yù Róng Gāo* (仙方玉容膏)

Xiān Fāng Yù Róng Gāo (仙方玉容膏) is a natural ointment that is neither greasy nor powdery. It is a technologically sophisticated extraction that is refined from *lú huì* (Aloe) and *huáng qí* (Radix Astragali).

Lü and his colleagues used it to treat pruritus in 126 cases, other ointments for random comparison.

Results: healed rate 53.97%, effective rate 29.37%, the total effective rate was 95.24%, which was obviously higher than comparison group ($P<0.01$), no adverse effect discerned.

Experimental studies showed *Xiān Fāng Yù Róng Gāo* (仙方玉容膏) had anti-inflammatory actions. It could inhibit swelling of the ear auricle caused by methylbenzene, as well as capillary permeability increased by the injection of histamine phosphate of rats. It also had anti-itching actions. Studies showed it could raise the itch threshold of the cavia cobaya to beta-imidazolyle thylamine160.0±101.29μg, while the *Jié Ěr Yīn* (洁尔阴) group was 220.50±16.68μg($P<0.05, P<0.01$). [35]

(2) Clinical and Experimental Studies of *Shén Míng Bái Gāo* (神明白膏) on the Ancient Formula Dunhuang in Treating Pruritus Senilis

Set up a treatment group of 100 cases, comparison group (999 *Pí Yán Píng Ruǎn Gāo* 皮炎平软膏) 30 cases, both were applied on affected parts for 1 month.

Results: the treatment group healed rate was 46%, the total effective rate was 92%; comparison group healed rate was 17%, the total effective rate was 67%. There was significant deviation between treatment group and the comparison group ($P<0.01$).

Experimental studies showed *Shén Míng Bái Gāo* (神 明 白 膏) had anti-inflammatory and relieving itching actions. There were no irritating or hypersensitive responses seen, nor side effects when applied locally. Conclusion: It was safe to use *Shén Míng Bái Gāo* (神 明 白 膏), and therapeutic effect can be achieved in treating alleviating pruritus senilis. [36]

(3) Observation of the Anti-itching and Antibacterial Actions of *Sāo Yǎng Líng Xiāng Lù* (瘙痒灵香露)

Observe an antibacterial experiment of the external product (includes *huáng bǎi* (Cortex Phellodendri Chinensis), *kǔ shēn* (Radix Sophorae Flavescentis), *dì fū zǐ* (Fructus Kochiae), *dú huó* (Radix Angelicae Pubescentis), *xì xīn* (Radix et Rhizoma Asari), *zhāng nǎo* (Camphora)) by successive dilution.

Results: The product had strong inhibitory actions on Staphylococcus aureus, aeruginosus Bacillus and Bacillus coli and had stronger action to inhibit Staphylococcus aureus.

Conclusions: The actions of the product dispelled wind to dry dampness, removed heat and toxins, killed parasites to relieve itching. Therefore it had unique therapeutic effects in treating eczema, dermatitis and pruritus due to wind-heat and dampness. [37]

REFERENCES

[1] Chen Hui-shi. Differentiation and Exploration of Cutaneous Pruritus (皮肤瘙痒症辨治探析). *Liaoning Journal of Traditional Chinese Medicine* (辽宁中医杂志). 2004, 31(11): 934.

[2] Wang Yu, Ye Hui. Insights from Treating Pruritus by Chinese Medicine (中医辨治皮肤瘙痒症的体会). *Journal of Liaoning College of Traditional Chinese Medicine* (辽宁中医学院学报). 2005, 7(3): 250.

[3] Han Yan-xia. Treatment with Syndrome Differentiation of 60 Cases of Pruritus Senilis (老年性皮肤瘙痒症辨证论治60例). *Chinese Journal of Gerontology* (中国老年学杂志), 2005, 25(5) :610.

[4] Tang De-mu, Fang Li-hua. *Yǎng Xuè Rùn Fū Tāng* Treating 60 Cases of Pruritus Senilis (养血润肤汤治疗老年性皮肤瘙痒症 60 例). *Journal of Anhui Traditional Chinese Medical College* (安徽中医学院学报). 1997, 16(3): 27.

[5] Guo Yi-wen, Huang Ge-ning, Pang Xin-li. Clinical Research on *Jiǔ Xiān Tāng* Treating Male Pruritus Senilis (韭仙汤治疗男性老年皮肤瘙痒症的临床研究). *Heibei Journal of Traditional Chinese Medicine* (河北中医). 2005, 27(5): 331.

[6] Gao Feng, Wang Qiang, Li Tie-nan. Observation of Therapeutic Effect of Blood-enriching and *Rùn Fū Zhǐ Yǎng Tāng* Treating Pruritus Senilis (润肤止痒汤治疗老年性皮肤瘙痒症疗效观察). *Chinese Journal of Dermatovenereology of Integrated Traditional And Western Medicine* (中国中西医结合皮肤性病学杂志). 2005, 4(3): 187.

[7] Sun Jia-cai. *Quán Xiē Zhǐ Yǎng Tāng* Treating Pruritus Senilis (全蝎止痒汤治疗老年性皮肤瘙痒症). *Clinical Journal of Anhui Traditional Chinese Medicine* (安徽中医临床杂志). 1998, 10(5): 332.

[8] Zhang Zi-fu. Modified *Guì Zhī Tāng* Treating 58 Cases of Pruritus Senilis (桂枝汤加味治疗老年性皮肤瘙痒 58 例). *Gansu Journal of Traditional Chinese Medicine* (甘肃中医). 1997, 10 (5): 18.

[9] Ma Lan. Observation of Therapeutic Effect of *Yǎng Xuè Rùn Fū Yǐn* for Treating Pruritus Senilis (养血润肤饮治疗老年性皮肤瘙痒症疗效观察). *Chinese Journal of Integrated Traditional and Western Medicine* (中国中西医结合杂志). 1997, 17(6): 375.

[10] Wang Cai-xiu, Zhao Li. Differentiation and Treatment of 20 Cases of Stubborn Pruritus Ani (顽固性肛门瘙痒症 20 例辨证治疗). *Journal of Traditional Chinese Medicine* (中医杂志). 1997, 38(10): 620.

[11] Zhang Shu-guang, Zhang Xiu-zhi. *Bǔ Xīn Tāng* for Treating 72 Cases of Pruritus Vulvae Senilis (补心汤治疗老年性外阴瘙痒症 72 例). *Shanxi Journal of Traditional Chinese Medicine* (山西中医). 1998, 4(1): 17.

[12] Lei Hong-ju. Clinic Observation of *Yǎng Xuè Róu Gān Huà Yū Tāng* for Treating 62 Cases of Pruritus Senilis (养血柔肝化瘀汤治疗老年性皮肤瘙痒症 62 例临床观察). *Chinese Journal of Dermatovenereology of Integrated Traditional And Western Medicine* (中国中西医结合皮肤性病学杂志). 2004, 3(1): 36-37.

[13] Ye Xing-ming, Zhang Chun-hui. *Dāng Guī Yǐn Zi* Primarily for Treating 78 Cases of Pruritus Senilis (当归饮子为主治疗老年性皮肤瘙痒 78 例). *Fujian Journal of Traditional Chinese Medicine* (福建中医药). 2001, 32(3): 431.

[14] Wang He-ping, Zhang Yang. Modified *Dāng Guī Yǐn Zi* for Treating 36 Cases of Pruritus Senilis (加味当归饮子治疗老年性皮肤瘙痒症 36 例). *Information of Traditional Chinese Medicine* (中医药信息). 2001, 18(2): 371.

[15] Zhang Guo-an, Yang Jing-jian. *Xuè Fēng Tāng* for Treating 52 Cases of Pruritus (血风汤治疗皮肤瘙痒症 52 例). *Hunan Journal of Traditional Chinese Medicine* (湖南中医杂志), 2000. 16 (1): 421.

[16] Yang Xue-jing. *Rùn Fū Zhǐ Yǎng Tāng* for Treating 30 Cases of Pruritus Senilis (润肤止痒汤治疗老年性皮肤瘙痒症 30 例). *Chinese Practical of Rural Doctor* (中国乡村医生杂志). 2001, (7): 42.

[17] Liu Zong-yan, Liu Cai-ying. *Dān Jī Yín Qiào Yǐn* for Treating 80 Cases of Pruritus (丹鸡银翘饮治疗皮肤瘙痒症 80 例). *Inner Mongol Journal of Traditional Chinese Medicine* (内蒙古中医药). 2001, (2): 71.

[18] Hu Zhi-fang, Xue Yu-shu. Created *Èr Chóng Sì Wù Tāng* for Treating 15 Cases of Pruritus Senilis (自拟二虫四物汤治疗老年皮肤瘙痒症 30 例). *Journal of Sichuan Traditional Chinese Medicine* (四川中医). 2000, 18(9): 501.

[19] Yin Chuan-kai, Li Wan-ping. *Dāng Guī Yǐn Zi Hé Sì Zhòng Tāng* for Treating 48 Cases of Pruritus Senilis (当归饮子合四重汤治疗老年皮肤瘙痒症 48 例). *Forum on traditional Chinese Medicine* (国医论坛). 2000, 15(4): 301.

[20] Xu Xiu-rong. Observation of Therapeutic Effects of *Biàn Tōng Guī Pí Tāng* for Treating Pruritus Senilis (变通归脾汤治疗老年性皮肤瘙痒症疗效观察). *Journal of Chinese Physician* (中国临床医生). 2001, 29(6): 411.

[21] Zhan Bo-xi. *Míng Fán Kǔ Jiāo Xūn Xǐ Jì* for Treating 68 Cases of Cutaneous

Pruritus Cutanea (明矾苦椒熏洗剂治疗风瘙痒 68 例). *The Chinese Journal of Dermatovenereology* (中国皮肤性病学杂志). 1996, 10(6): 371.

[22] Pan Yu-wei, Zhang Si-hu. Recent Developments in Chinese Medicine Treating Pruritus Senilis (老年性皮肤瘙痒症中医治疗近况). *Jiangsu Journal of Traditional Chinese Medicine* (江苏中医药). 2004, 25(11): 64-66.

[23] Song Guang-ying. Observation of Clinical Application of *Shū Fū Săn* in Dermatology (舒肤散在皮肤科的临床应用观察). *Modern Journal of Integrated Traditional Chinese and Western Medicine* (现代中西医结合杂志). 2004, 13(6): 770.

[24] Wang Wei-ping, Jia Hai-yan, Jia Chao-ying. *Liáng Xuè Huó Xuè Zhǐ Yăng Fāng* for Treating 25 Cases of Pruritus Senilis by Applying on Bellybutton (凉血活血止痒方敷脐治疗老年瘙痒症 25 例). *Journal of External Therapy of Traditional Chinese Medicine* (中医外治杂志). 2002, 11(5): 41.

[25] Li Jian-lan, Han Jian-lan. Treating 38 Cases of Pruritus by Acupuncture Primarily (针刺为主治疗皮肤瘙痒症 38 例). *Chinese Acupuncture and Moxibustion* (中国针灸). 2001, 21(2): 122.

[26] Yang Chang-ming, Mao Jing-lie, Yu Ju. Observation of Therapeutic Effect of Treating Pruritus Senilis by Acupuncture (针灸治疗老年性皮肤瘙痒症疗效观察). *Chinese Acupuncture and Moxibustion* (中国针灸). 2002, 22(7): 459.

[27] Tang Guo-lian. Clinical Observation of 40 Cases of Pruritus Senilis (针灸治疗老年性瘙痒病 40 例临床观察). *Chinese Acupuncture and Moxibustion* (中国针灸). 1996, 12 (10): 42.

[28] He Jing-guo, Xu Ai-zhen. Pyonex Matching Chinese Medicinals to Treat 65 Cases of Pruritus Senilis (梅花针配合中药治疗老年性皮肤瘙痒症 65 例). *Hubei Journal of Traditional Chinese Medicine* (湖北中医杂志). 1996, 122(3): 31.

[29] Xu Shan-ying. Clinical Observation of Moxa-wool Moxibustion for Treating 72 Cases of Pruritus Ani (艾灸治疗肛门瘙痒症 72 例临床观察). *Journal of Beijing Traditional Chinese Medicine* (北京中医). 1997, 3: 30.

[30] Liu Shi-zhong. Needle Implant in Ear Acupoints to Treat 44 Cases of Pruritus Vulvae (耳穴埋针治疗阴痒 44 例). *Chinese Acupuncture and Moxibustion* (中国针灸). 1996, 16 (6): 37.

[31] Liu Min. Differentiation and Treatment of 80 Cases of Pruritus Vulvae by Ear Acupuncture (耳针为主辨证治疗阴痒 80 例). *Journal of Clinical Acupuncture and Moxibustion* (针灸临床杂志). 1997, 13(10): 24.

[32] Zhang Jie, Zhang Jian-hua. Ear Pressure Therapy Treating Pruritus (耳穴贴压治疗皮肤瘙痒症). *Chinese Acupuncture and Moxibustion* (中国针灸). 2002, 22(12): 827.

[33] Zhang Yan-li. Needling Matching Cupping Treating Pruritus (针刺配合拔罐治疗皮肤瘙痒). *Chinese Acupuncture and Moxibustion* (中国针灸). 2002, 22(12): 826.

[34] Liu Jian-xin. Back Needling Matching Cupping Treating Pruritus (背部叩刺加拔罐治疗皮肤瘙痒症). *Chinese Acupuncture and Moxibustion* (中国针灸). 2002, 22(12): 826.

[35] Lü Ming-zhuang, He Zhi-guang. Clinical and Empirical Studies on *Xiān Fāng Yù Róng Gāo* (仙方玉容膏治疗皮肤瘙痒症的临床和实验研究). *Yunnan Journal of Traditional Chinese Medicine and Materia Medica* (云南中医中药杂志). 1998, 19(4): 31-33.

[36] Zhang Shi-qing, Xia Zhi-bo, Zhu Xue-yi. Clinical and Empirical Studies on Dunhuang Ancient Formula *Shén Míng Bái Gāo* Treating Pruritus Senilis (敦煌古方神明白膏治疗老年性皮肤瘙痒病的临床疗效与实验研究). *China Association of Traditional Chinese Medicine* (中医药学刊). 2003, 21(1): 86-88.

[37] Lei Xiao-ming, Liu Wen-tai, Li Li-hua. Mechanism Studies of *Sāo Yǎng Líng Xiāng Lù* (观察瘙痒灵香露止痒机制的研究). *Chinese Journal of Basic Medicine in Traditional Chinese Medicine* (中国中医基础医学杂志). 2005, 11(9): 668-672.

Index by Disease Names and Symptoms

Index by Chinese Medicinals and Formulas

D

R

General Index

D

G

H

I

J

K

L

M

Notes

图书在版编目（CIP）数据

中医临床实用系列：银屑病与皮肤瘙痒症（英文）/ 卢传坚等主编．—北京：人民卫生出版社，2007.10

ISBN 978-7-117-09242-5

Ⅰ．中…　Ⅱ．卢…　Ⅲ．①银屑病－中医治疗法－英文②瘙痒－中医治疗法－英文　Ⅳ．R275.986.3　R275.983

中国版本图书馆 CIP 数据核字（2007）第 141282 号

中医临床实用系列：银屑病与皮肤瘙痒症（英文）

主　　编：卢传坚　禤国维
出版发行：人民卫生出版社（中继线 +8610-6761-6688）
地　　址：中国北京市丰台区方庄芳群园三区 3 号楼
邮　　编：100078
网　　址：http://www.pmph.com
E - mail：pmph @ pmph.com
发　　行：zzg@pmph.com.cn
购书热线：+8610-6769-1034（电话及传真）
开　　本：787×1092　1/16
版　　次：2007 年 10 月第 1 版　2007 年 10 月第 1 版第 1 次印刷
标准书号：ISBN 978-7-117-09242-5/R・9243